Designing Network Security for a Microsoft® Windows® Server 2003 Network

Project Lab Manual

Exam 70-298

Designing Network Security for a Microsoft® Windows® Server 2003 Network

Project Lab Manual
Exam 70-298

First Edition

Kenneth C. Laudon, Series Designer
Frank Miller, MCSE, MCSA

The Azimuth Interactive MCSE/MCSA Team
Carol G. Traver, Series Editor
Kenneth Rosenblatt
Robin L. Pickering
Russell Polo
David Langley
Megan Miller
Brian Hill, MCSE, MCSA
Stacey McBrine, MCSE, MCSA
Richard Watson, MCSE
Brien Posey, MCSE
Tim Oliwiak, MCSE, MCT
David Lundell, MCSE, MCT
L. Ward Ulmer, MCSE, MCT
Wale Soyinka, MCP
Simon Sykes-Wright, MCSE
David W. Tschanz, MCSE
Russell Jones, MCSE
Pete Grondin, MCSA
Lenny Bailes
Mark Maxwell

PEARSON
Prentice Hall

Upper Saddle River, New Jersey, 07458

Senior Vice President/Publisher: Natalie Anderson
Executive Acquisitions Editor: Stephanie Wall
Marketing Manager: Sarah Davis
Project Manager, Editorial: Laura Burgess
Manager, Print Production: Christy Mahon
Production Editor & Buyer: Carol O'Rourke
Composition: Azimuth Interactive, Inc.
Quality Assurance: Specialized Composition, Inc.
Printer/Binder: Banta, Harrisonburg

PEARSON
Prentice Hall

10 9 8 7 6 5 4 3 2 1
ISBN 0-13-146684-4

To our families,
for their love, patience,
and inspiration.

Brief Contents

Contents

Preface

The purpose of this Project Lab Manual is to provide you, the student, with another opportunity to review Windows Server 2003 concepts and skills, and to apply them to situations that you are likely to encounter on the job. The Prentice Hall Certification Series textbooks contain a great deal of conceptual and hands-on material. The Prentice Hall Certification Series Project Lab Manuals are designed to give you an opportunity to put those concepts and skills to work in a variety of different real-world on-the-job situations, and to understand the textbook contents in greater depth.

The Project Lab Manuals are organized in the same two-page highly illustrated format with conceptual material and instructions on the left-hand page, and screenshots and conceptual diagrams on the right-hand page. The Lessons in the Project Lab Manuals follow the Lessons in the textbook. Each Project Lab Manual Lesson is composed of a number of projects that reinforce the concepts and skills taught in the accompanying textbooks.

Project Lab Manual Lesson Contents

The Project Lab Manual Lessons have a number of elements designed to speed your learning and help you understand key concepts and skills.

Introductory Page: Each Lesson begins with an introductory page that reviews the key concepts and skills that you will be asked to apply in the lesson.

Scenario: Each Lesson has a brief scenario that describes the setting in which the projects take place. These scenarios provide you with a sense of how the concepts and skills that you have learned in the book are used in realistic business settings.

Project/Objective Table: Each Lesson includes a table that lists the Lesson projects and the corresponding exam objective supported. Where the project relates to a basic understanding of the subject matter, this is referred to as "Basic knowledge." You will always know how a project relates to MCSE exam requirements.

General Requirements: At the beginning of each Lesson, there is a description of the hardware and software that you will need to complete the projects in the Lesson.

Project's Exam Objective: For each project there is a description of the specific MCSE exam objective supported by the project.

Overview: Each project presents a specific assignment that builds on the Lesson's main scenario.

Learning Objective: Each project includes a specific learning objective that describes what you will be able to do after completing the project.

Specific Requirements: A list of specific requirements for each project is provided.

Estimated Completion Time: For each project, there is an estimated time for completion based on the experience of MCSE professionals and instructors in colleges and training institutes. You should use these estimates only as a guide because your actual completion times will depend on your prior experience with Windows Server 2003.

Project Steps: Each project includes a set of step-by-step instructions for completing the project. These instructions are similar to those in the main textbook, but often differ because new options and pathways may be explored in the Project Lab Manuals.

Tips: Throughout the Project Lab Manuals you will find Tips and Cautions that offer you suggestions or comments about completing the project and working with Windows Server 2003.

Graphics and Illustrations: As you can expect from the Prentice Hall Certification Series, there are many screenshots and conceptual graphics provided that show you how the software should look at various points in the project. These are intended to familiarize you with the Windows Server 2003 environment and assure you that you are on the right track.

Quality Assurance

We have made every effort to ensure that the Project Lab Manuals are written to the same quality standards as the main textbook. The Project Lab Manuals are written by MCSE professionals with many years of real-world experience. The initial instructions and scenarios are then reviewed by independent technical editors who test each project, and each step. These results are then verified by the MCSE team at Azimuth and the Series Designer and Editor. The end result is a product that students and instructors can understand and trust.

Notice

The projects in the Project Lab Manuals have been built using the most recent release of Windows Server 2003 and Windows XP Professional software. Your school or other institution may be using an earlier release of the software, or its environment may differ in some respects from the environment in which the projects were built. At times, these variations in environment and service packs can cause variations in the progression of steps and screenshots so that a screenshot in the book does not precisely match the screen you may be looking at. If this should occur, please report this to the authors at the Web site for this book.

LESSON

1 Analyzing Business and Technical Requirements

Secure network design has never been more critical that it is today. Knowledgeable organizations understand that a secure computing infrastructure is a vital business resource, and that a secure network is a critical component of that resource.

Windows Server 2003 is designed to provide a secure network platform. However, there are no "one size fits all" security solutions. Designing an appropriate security solution means you must understand:

- How the business is organized
- Short- and long-term business goals
- Management and user commitment to security
- Willingness and ability to invest in security solutions

One advantage you have today is that most organizations know that they have experienced security breaches in the past and understand the potential impact. This makes decision makers more open to the need to secure network resources, seeing the process as an investment in the future.

You must understand an organization's needs before you can propose solutions. The first step in security design is detailed security analysis. You can get an initial overview from the organization's Mission statement (the "who" and "why" of the business) and vision statement (its business goals).

Several factors must be considered in a security design, including:

- **Cost:** Internal and contracted personnel, hardware investments, software investments, total cost of ownership (TCO), and assets to be protected.
- **Legal requirements:** Local, national, and international security laws and regulations, as applicable to the business.
- **End-user impact:** Specifying security through policy and procedures, education in security requirements, and enforcing security through network tools.
- **Risk:** Identifying perceived risks and risk management requirements.
- **Interoperability:** Compatibility with legacy and future hardware and software.
- **Maintainability and scalability:** Cost and effort required to maintain security solutions.

Success of a security design depends on management and end-user buy-in and acceptance. Users are often informed and educated through written policies and procedures, which must be written in language that is easily understood by users. Security procedures should require as little direct user effort as possible, focusing on security that can be enforced through hardware or software.

A major part of any network security design is business data. You must identify:

- What data is important and why
- Who (internally) should have access to the data
- Who (externally) should have access to the data
- The data you are required to protect (by law and regulation) and the level of protection required

Identify, organize, and classify all business data. Analyze data, current data use, and projected data requirements.

Security risks are inherent in organizations, with some risks built into the information technology (IT) department structure. Identify IT personnel, responsibilities, and access to sensitive data. Focus on key individuals, key responsibilities, reporting structures, and security boundaries.

Scenario

You are a security consultant brought in to head up a team designing security for Ready-Biz. Ready-Biz is a multinational manufacturing company. It is organized in three divisions along geographic lines, divided roughly as the United States and North America, European Union, and Pacific Rim. Each division is managed as a semi-autonomous entity.

The Ready-Biz enterprise network is organized as a Windows Active Directory forest containing three directory trees. In the United States, the parent domain is in the main office in Chicago, Illinois, with child domains in each of the major regional offices. Each location has at least two domain controllers. The company has recently upgraded all domain controllers to Windows Server 2003. The Chicago office also hosts two Web servers and an Exchange 2003 server providing mail support for most of the United States.

You are primarily responsible for the United States division, but will have limited oversight of and responsibility for coordination with the international divisions. You will develop an enterprise network security design. You must start by analyzing the current business structure and security requirements.

Lesson 1 Analyzing Business and Technical Requirements

Project	*Exam 70-298 Objective*
1.1 Balancing Business Objectives with Technical Design	**Analyze business requirements for designing security. Considerations include existing policies and procedures, sensitivity of data, cost, legal requirements, end-user impact, interoperability, maintainability, scalability, and risk.**
1.2. Introducing Security Policies and Procedures	**Analyze business requirements for designing security. Considerations include existing policies and procedures, sensitivity of data, cost, legal requirements, end-user impact, interoperability, maintainability, scalability, and risk**. Analyze existing security policies and procedures.
1.3. Organizing and Securing Data	**Analyze business requirements for designing security. Considerations include existing policies and procedures, sensitivity of data, cost, legal requirements, end-user impact, interoperability, maintainability, scalability, and risk. Analyze the organizational requirements for security data**. Analyze the security requirements for different types of data.
1.4 Analyzing Security Risks Within the IT Administration Structure	**Analyze business requirements for designing security. Considerations include existing policies and procedures, sensitivity of data, cost, legal requirements, end-user impact, interoperability, maintainability, scalability, and risk**. Analyze risks to security within the current IT administration structure and security practices.

General Requirements

There are no special requirements for this lesson. However, you may find it helpful to refer to Lesson 1 in your Prentice Hall Certification Series Exam 70-298 textbook for additional information about the topics covered by the projects in this lesson.

project 1.1

Balancing Business Objectives with Technical Design

exam objective

Analyze business requirements for designing security. Considerations include existing policies and procedures, sensitivity of data, cost, legal requirements, end-user impact, interoperability, maintainability, scalability, and risk.

overview

You must begin by identifying the security objectives that must be met and how they are balanced against business requirements **(Figure 1-1)**.

Learning objective

After completing this project, you will be able to identify keys areas of security analysis and available tools.

specific requirements

None

estimated completion time

15 minutes

project steps

1. Identify key areas that must be included in your security design. For each of these areas, suggest possible sources for the information you need.
2. Describe how the Microsoft Operations Framework (MOF) can aid in risk analysis and risk management planning **(Figure 1-2)**.
3. Prepare a document setting out general guidelines for the type of information you will need for the lead consultants in the international divisions to be able to complete your security design.

Figure 1-1 Business requirements impact the security design

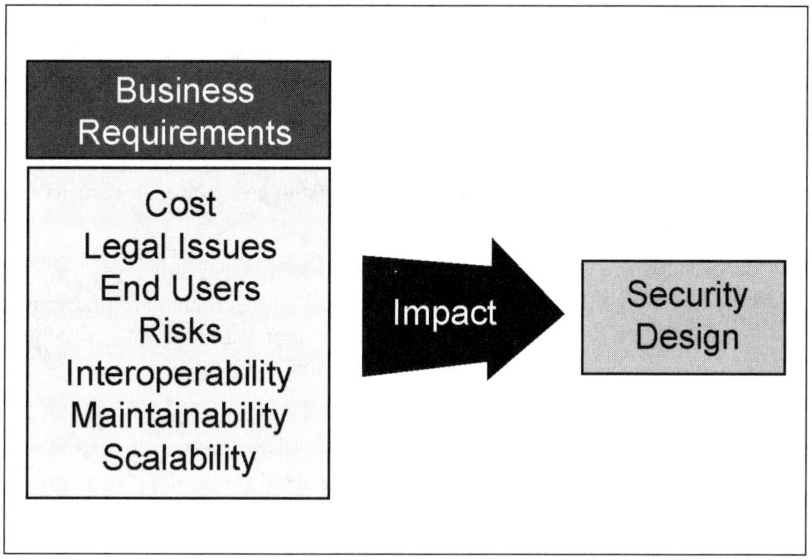

Figure 1-2 Microsoft Operations Framework (MOF) risk model

- Step 1: Identifying Risks in Operations
- Step 2: Analyzing and Prioritizing Risks
- Step 3: Planning and Scheduling Risk Actions
- Step 4: Tracking and Reporting Risks
- Step 5: Controlling Risks
- Step 6: Learning from Risk

project 1.2

Introducing Security Policies and Procedures

exam objective

Analyze business requirements for designing security. Considerations include existing policies and procedures, sensitivity of data, cost, legal requirements, end-user impact, interoperability, maintainability, scalability, and risk. Analyze existing security policies and procedures.

overview

You must identify the role of policies and procedures in security analysis and in implementing a security design.

The primary means through which Ready-Biz currently implements network security is through written security policies. Policy documents are distributed to end users on a regular basis. New policy documents are distributed each month, whether or not there have been any changes to the policies in effect **(Figure 1-3)**.

Users complain that the language used in the security policies is confusing, and that the instructions often seem contradictory. Users are not allowed to ask network administrators to explain network policies, but must instead send information requests to the IT department in writing **(Figure 1-4)**.

Most security decisions are left up to each regional office. Regional offices are expected to provide the Chicago office with copies of their current security policies.

learning objective

After completing this project, you will be more familiar with key issues relating to policies and procedures.

specific requirements

None

estimated completion time

15 minutes

project steps

1. Before analyzing current policies and procedures, identify areas where policies and procedures fail to be implemented by users.
2. Explain why security procedures that can be implemented through network security are preferred over written security policies.
3. Identify reasons why employees are typically a company's biggest security risk.

Figure 1-3 Why security policy and procedures fail

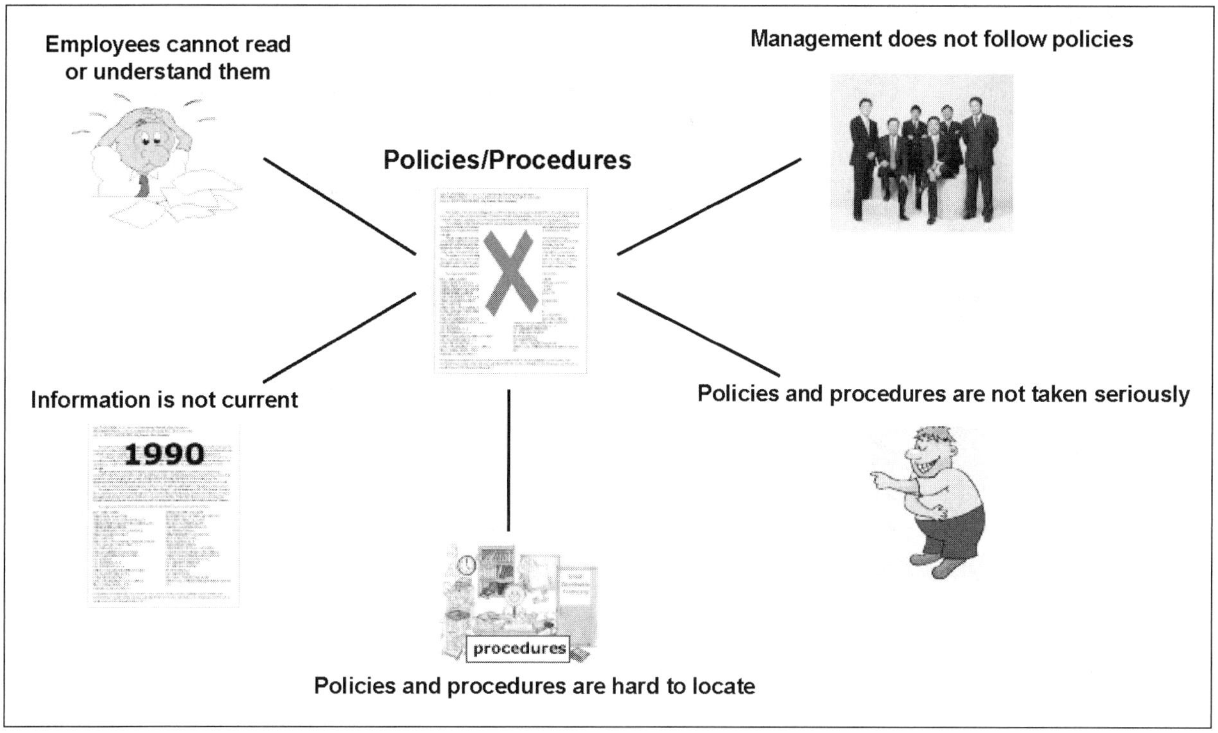

Figure 1-4 Security design impact on users

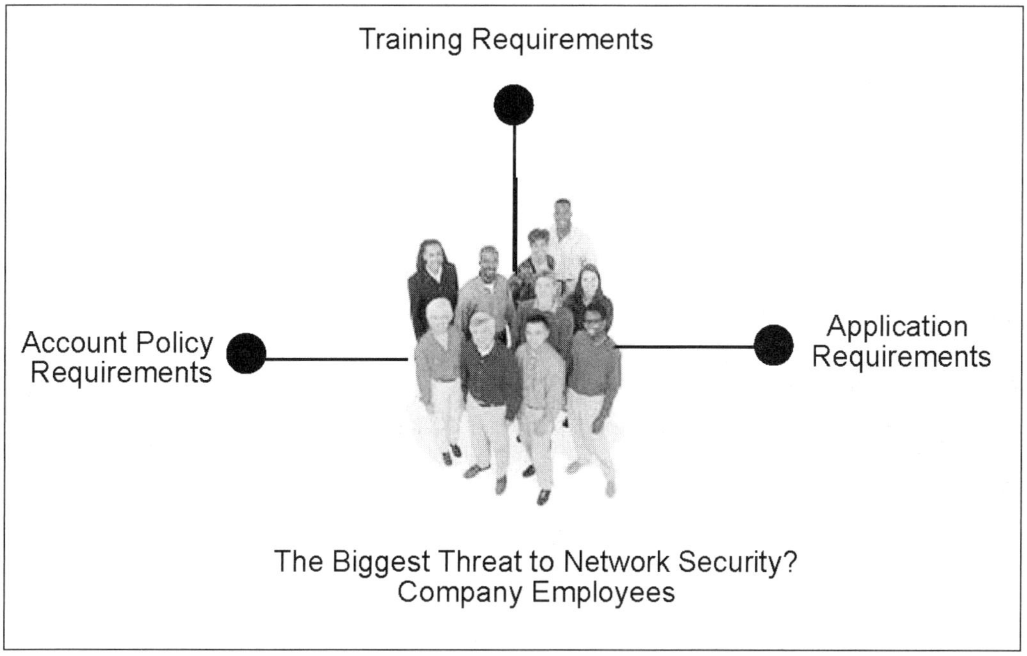

project 1.3

Organizing and Securing Data

exam objective

Analyze business requirements for designing security. Considerations include existing policies and procedures, sensitivity of data, cost, legal requirements, end-user impact, interoperability, maintainability, scalability, and risk. Analyze the organizational requirements for securing data. Analyze the security requirements for different types of data.

overview

All current company data is referred to by the blanket term of "company confidential." Major categories of data **(Figure 1-5)** include the following:

- Product inventories
- Raw material costs
- Product design documents
- Sales and cost of sales information
- Price lists and discount policies
- List prices
- Current customers
- Product descriptions and sales brochures
- Employee and related human resource information

Data storage is poorly organized, left primarily to the users generating and using the data. Each region is responsible for its own data. There is no central data repository.

learning objective

After completing this project, you will be able to identify data structures and the importance of organizing data.

specific requirements

None

estimated completion time

10 minutes

project steps

1. What data must be protected by law or regulation? What data is critical to business operations?
2. What are justifications for centralizing data in one location **(Figure 1-6)**? What are potential drawbacks of centralizing data?
3. Categorize the Ready-Biz data as Confidential, Public, Private, or Sensitive.

Figure 1-5 Examples of data categories

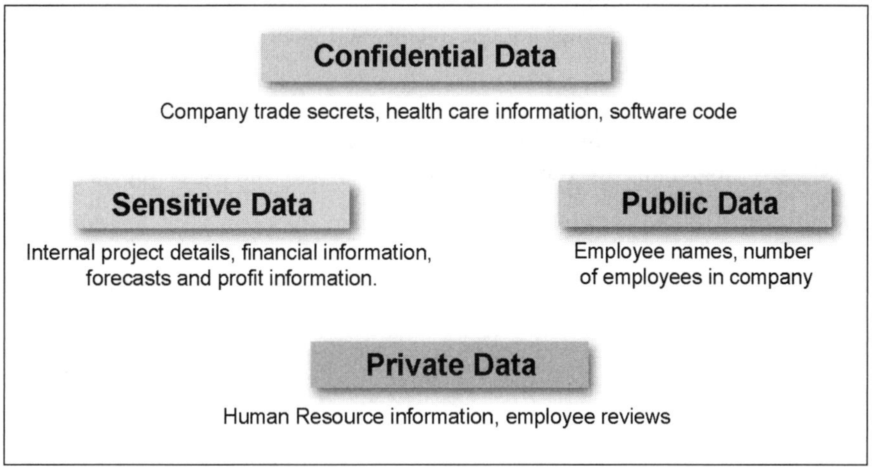

Figure 1-6 Justifications for protecting data

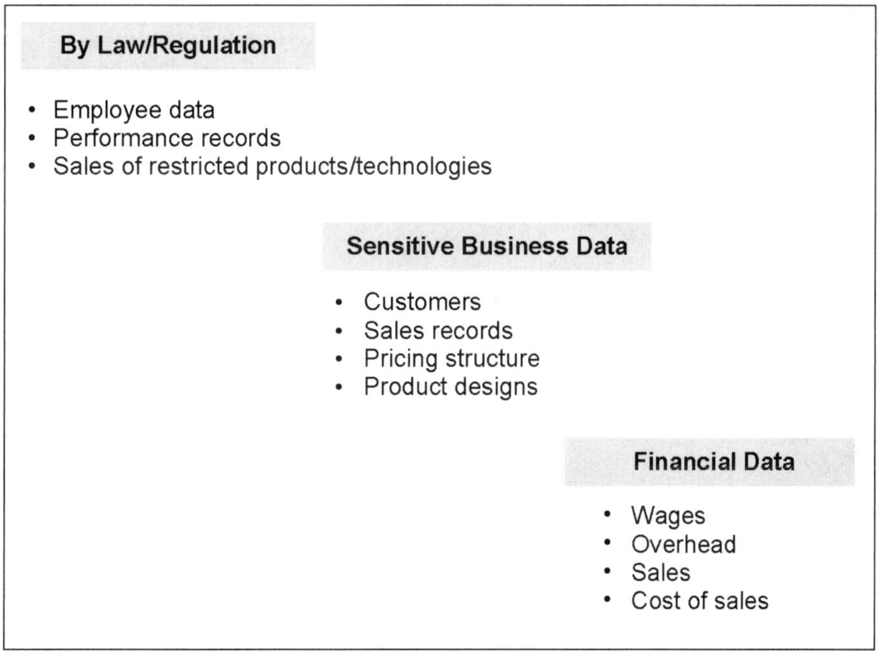

project 1.4

Analyzing Security Risks Within the IT Administration Structure

exam objective

Analyze business requirements for designing security. Considerations include existing policies and procedures, sensitivity of data, cost, legal requirements, end-user impact, interoperability, maintainability, scalability, and risk. Analyze risks to security within the current IT administration structure and security practices.

overview

You must identify potential IT structure risks that you must watch for and identify. You do not know if any of these risks are present in the Ready-Biz IT department structure. Each region maintains its own IT department. This model is repeated throughout the enterprise (**Figure 1-7**).

learning objective

After completing this project, you will be able to identify the potential security risks inherent in an IT structure.

specific requirements

None

estimated completion time

10 minutes

project steps

1. What types of documents would assist you in determining how the IT department is structured and which individuals are department decision makers?
2. Prepare a short memo justifying consolidation of regional IT departments under one managing director (**Figure 1-8**).
3. What are the management boundaries within the United States? Internationally?

Figure 1-7 Sample organizational chart

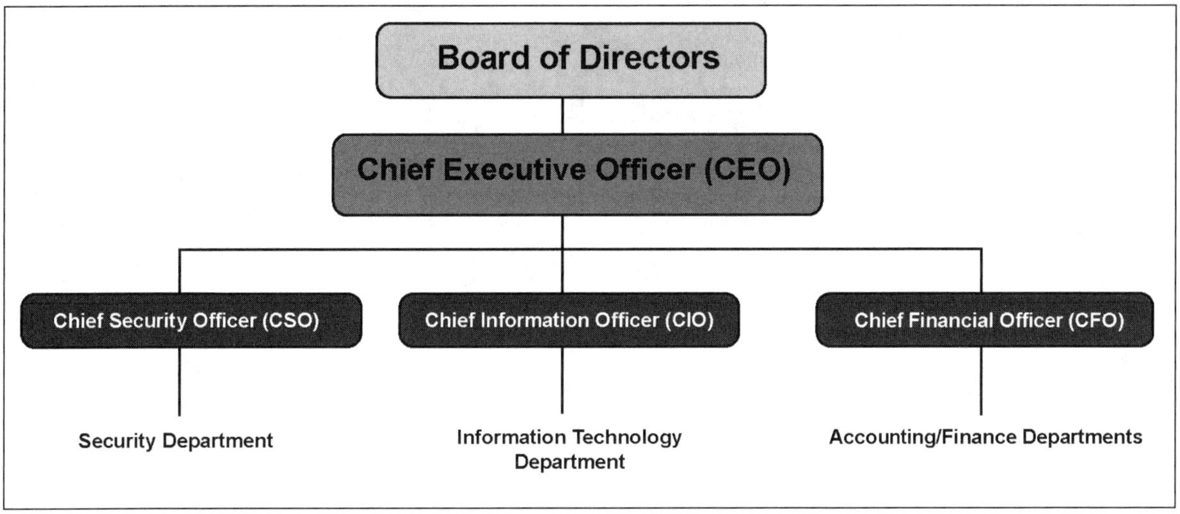

Figure 1-8 Possible IT responsibilities

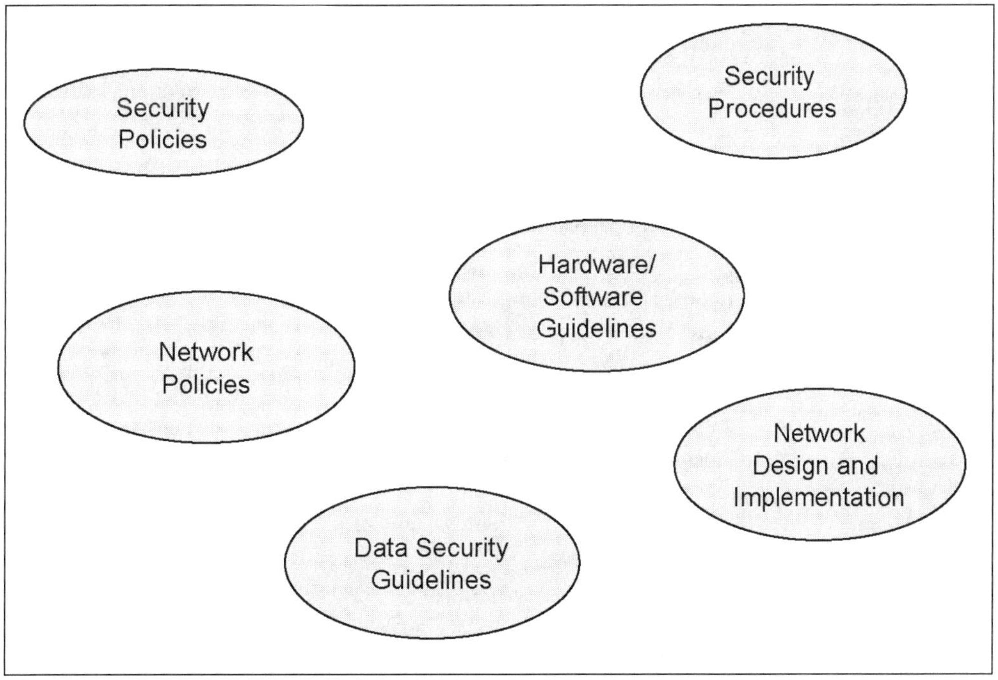

LESSON

2 Planning a Framework for Designing and Implementing Security

In Lesson 1, you were introduced to fundamental concepts relating to security analysis and identifying potential security risks. This lesson continues the initial security planning process by introducing security plan components designed to help you recognize and deal with these threats.

Threat modeling is the process of identifying and understanding vulnerabilities. This is a team-based process requiring a mix of technical skills. The STRIDE model is the current standard model for identifying the following common threats:

- **Spoofing:** Attack through impersonation.
- **Tampering:** Attack through data modification.
- **Repudiation:** Attack by disowning legitimate transactions.
- **Information disclosure:** Attack through unauthorized access to data.
- **Denial of Service (DoS) attack:** Attack by denying users access to resources.
- **Elevation of Privilege:** Attack by illegitimately obtaining administrative privileges.

Once you understand the potential vulnerabilities, you must determine how you will respond when security incidents occur. This is documented through incident response procedures and implemented through a Computer Security Incident Response Team (CSIRT). Typically, you will have multiple response procedures based on type and severity (critical level) of incidents. An incident response procedure should include:

- **Purpose statement:** Specifies procedure purpose
- **Scope:** Defines the area covered by procedure
- **Definition of incident:** Provides a description of the incident
- **Definition of roles:** Lists tasks and responsibilities, including CSIRT responsibilities
- **Classification of incidents/initial response:** Defines incident categories by critical level
- **Collection and protection of evidence:** Procedures for evidence gathering and chain of custody requirements
- **Documentation of incident:** Details of incident and CSIRT response, including any lessons learned from incident

An important part of protecting critical network resources from internal and external threats is the use of segmented networks. Network segmentation includes protecting "public" resources, such as Web services, isolating the internal network from the Internet, and isolating sensitive resources from the internal network.

Network segmentation is typically implemented through a mix of hardware and software resources. The segmentation model will be somewhat organization-specific.

Understanding that security incidents can and will occur means accepting the need for disaster recovery plans. Rank network resources by sensitivity and how critical they are to operational activities. This enables you to identify resources by relative priority and acceptable down time. Disaster recovery requirements include scheduled backup procedures, data recovery procedures, and operating system-specific automated recovery procedures.

Recovery priorities should be made available to all individuals involved in the recovery process, including end users. All procedures should be clearly documented as step-by-step, easy to follow processes.

Scenario

You are continuing to work with Ready-Biz in analyzing organizational security and designing reaction plans. Your responsibility is to help them identify their most critical vulnerabilities, the types of attacks that are most likely to occur, and the best ways to respond to the attacks. During this process, you are directly responsible for the United States division only, but may be called upon to provide advice and assistance to planning teams working with the other divisions.

Lesson 2 Planning a Framework for Designing and Implementing Security

Project	Exam 70-298 Objective
2.1 Predicting Threats from Internal and External Sources	**Design a framework for designing and implementing security. The framework should include prevention, detection, isolation, and recovery**. Predict threats to your network from internal and external sources.
2.2 Designing an Incident Response Process	**Design a framework for designing and implementing security. The framework should include prevention, detection, isolation, and recovery**. Design a process for responding to incidents.
2.3 Designing Segmented Networks	**Design a framework for designing and implementing security. The framework should include prevention, detection, isolation, and recovery**. Design segmented networks.
2.4 Recovering Services	**Design a framework for designing and implementing security. The framework should include prevention, detection, isolation, and recovery**. Design a process for recovering services.

General Requirements

There are no special requirements for this lesson. However, you may find it helpful to refer to Lesson 2 in your Prentice Hall Certification Series Exam 70-298 textbook for additional information about the topics covered by the projects in this lesson.

project 2.1

Predicting Threats from Internal and External Sources

exam objective

Design a framework for designing and implementing security. The framework should include prevention, detection, isolation, and recovery. Predict threats to your network from internal and external sources.

overview

Ready-Biz is aware that the company has experienced recent security incidents **(Table 2-1).** You are assigned a team that includes both management and employees to investigate how these incidents were able to occur, as well as identify other potential risks.

There is a prevailing corporate culture that the real threat is from external sources. Management staff wants to see a plan that almost exclusively addresses avoiding external attacks. Part of your job is convincing the management staff about the potential risk from internal attacks.

Learning objective

After completing this project, you will understand how to apply the STRIDE model to threat modeling.

specific requirements

None

estimated completion time

10 minutes

project steps

These questions address the security incidents described in Table 2-1.

1. Which threats are most likely the result of external attacks?
2. Which threats are most likely the result of internal attacks?
3. Based on what you know so far about the threats, prepare a short memo describing which threat time has resulted in the larger number of incidents and why this should be a concern.
4. Suggest Windows Server 2003 features that can help isolate the cause of the Elevation of Privilege incidents.

Table 2-1 STRIDE Threat Examples

Threat	Example
Spoofing	An individual uses e-mail addresses of users in Ready-Biz to send e-mail to customers. The threat isn't discovered until customers respond to the e-mails.
Tampering	An individual is directly modifying sales data in a SQL Server 2000 database to make it appear that some salespeople have better sales performance. It appears that warehouse inventory levels have been artificially reduced to match the false sales records. The errors are discovered during an end-of-quarter audit.
Repudiation	A customer complains about items received that were never ordered. A check of sales records verifies that the orders are on file, but the inside salesperson whose name is on the orders denies placing them.
Information disclosure	Inside salespeople were surprised one recent morning to find a report listing all inside and outside sales personnel, sales performance, and commission percentage. To say that there has been grumbling is an understatement.
Denial of Service (DoS)	The public Web server has been under intermittent attack, making is difficult for customers to access the Web site. The problem was discovered when a customer who usually places orders directly online calls to complain.
Elevation of Privilege	A department supervisor delegated administrator permissions over one department has somehow gained additional privileges and is making changes to user accounts throughout the organization. Authentication control and data access control are in shambles. Users complain about spontaneous password and access permission changes. The changes are happening most often to internal sales, order processing, and warehouse personnel.

project 2.2

Designing an Incident Response Process

exam objective

Design a framework for designing and implementing security. The framework should include prevention, detection, isolation, and recovery. Design a process for responding to incidents.

overview

Ready-Biz does not currently have a formal incident response program **(Figure 2-1)** in place nor follows accepted security awareness guidelines **(Figure 2-2)**. Instead, the company uses an informal "You found it, you fix it" model. Users are expected to contact network and IT personnel as necessary for assistance in fixing any problems that they discover.

There is also no formal reporting or follow-up in place. Reporting is typically through word-of-mouth. The network administration staff has started having weekly lunch meetings to discuss problems encountered during the week, incident status, and what was done to resolve the incident. The meeting is held in Chicago and staff members in other offices included through conference call, if included at all. Results of these staff meetings are not published outside of the network administration department.

learning objective

After completing this project, you will understand the importance of a formal incident response process and an identified Computer Security Incident Response Team (CSIRT).

specific requirements

None

estimated completion time

15 minutes

project steps

1. What are the major shortcomings of the current incident response process?
2. Why would it be difficult to prosecute anyone for illegal activities resulting in security incidents in the current system?
3. What are the primary justifications for documenting and reporting security incidents?
4. What procedures are currently in place that can be used as a basis for building an incident response team?
5. Prepare a short memo describing the importance of classifying potential incidents by critical level.

Figure 2-1 Incident response procedure components

- ✓ Purpose Statement
- ✓ Scope
- ✓ Definition of Incident
- ✓ Definition of Roles
- ✓ Classification of Incident/Initial Response
- ✓ Collection and Protection of Evidence
- ✓ Documentation of Incident

Figure 2-2 Security awareness guidelines

SECURITY AWARENESS

Communicate management guidelines to everyone

Keep security awareness training in front of employees at all times

Employees must understand security controls

Train employees to recognize intrusions

Train employees on how to respond to intrusions

project 2.3 Designing Segmented Networks

exam objective

Design a framework for designing and implementing security. The framework should include prevention, detection, isolation, and recovery. Design segmented networks.

overview

You are provided with the network development plans for the next six months. The public Web servers will be remaining in Chicago only, but will be increased to four servers using load balancing. Each office will be setting up a Web server for that office's internal use. The mail organization is being expanded to place an Exchange 2003 mail server in each location.

You've been asked to prepare a segmented network design **(Figure 2-3)** for the Chicago office that can be used as the basis for network organization in the other offices. The United States division will migrate to a new configuration first, and if successful, the model will be carried across to the other offices.

In reviewing the overall business plan, you see that the company is planning to implement commerce servers as a way of automating business-to-business (B2B) communications, both with customers and suppliers. These were omitted from the hardware projections you were given.

learning objective

After completing this project, you will understand the need for network segmentation and develop segmented network designs.

specific requirements

None

estimated completion time

10 minutes

project steps

1. What servers and resources would you place in a perimeter network?
2. What servers and resources would you place on the internal network?
3. Refer to the scenario at the beginning of Lesson 1, if necessary. What resources might you place on a secure LAN segment in the Chicago office?
4. Justify the need for a perimeter network in each of the offices.

Figure 2-3 Segmented network examples

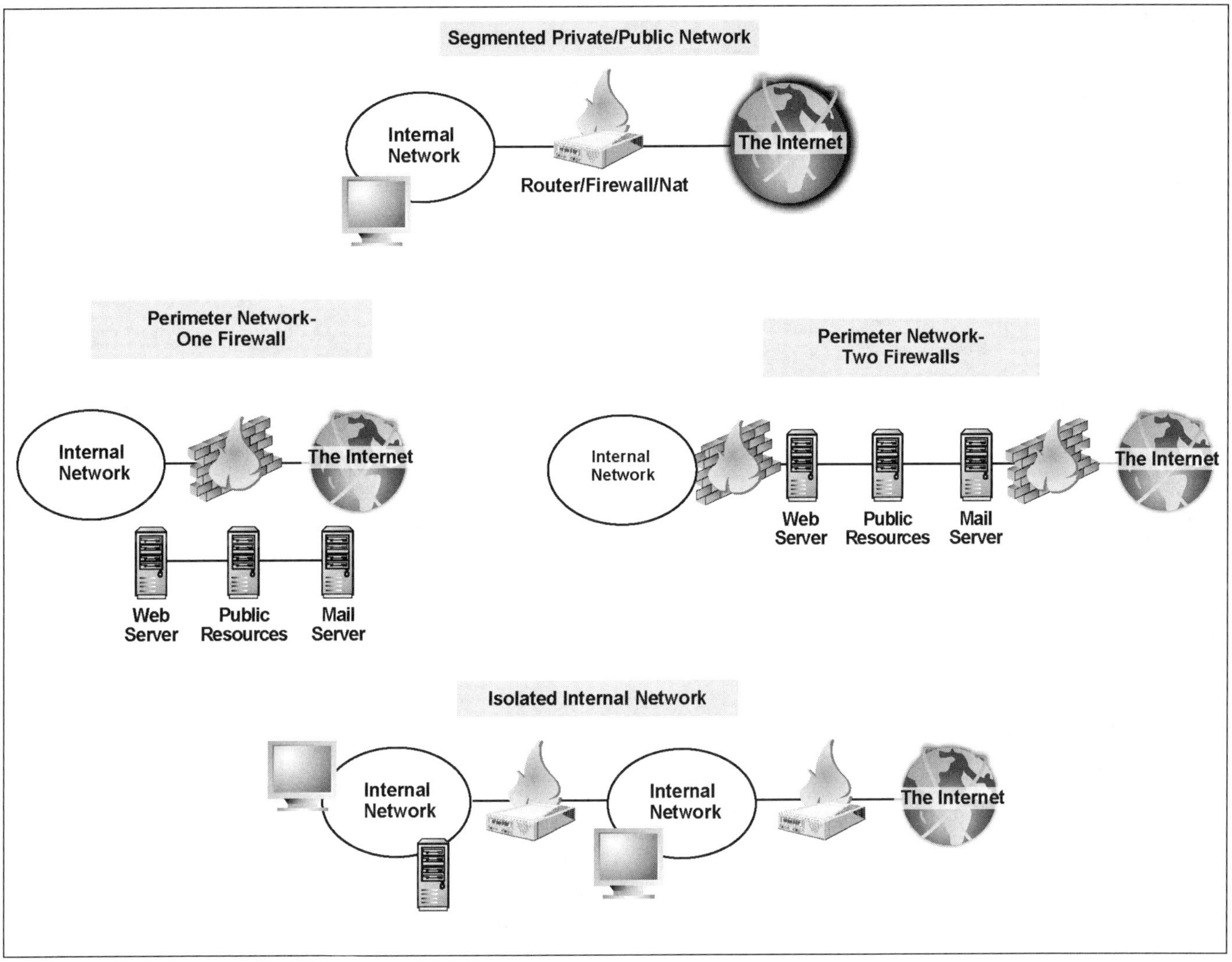

project 2.4

Recovering Services

exam objective

Design a framework for designing and implementing security. The framework should include prevention, detection, isolation, and recovery. Design a process for recovering services.

overview

Individual users are responsible for data backups for data on their own computers. Each department is responsible for departmental servers with the exception of shared file servers, database servers, mail servers, and Web servers. These are the responsibility of network support.

Ready-Biz has no disaster recovery plan **(Figure 2-4)** in place. Working with the management team, you have categories of activities within the companies such as:

- Sales
- Marketing and advertisement
- Warehouse and shipping
- Research and development
- Receiving and manufacturing
- Accounting
- Operations

You need to identify business-critical operations and systems, and potential disasters **(Figure 2-5)**, and then develop a disaster recovery plan.

learning objective

After completing this project, you will be more familiar with disaster recovery fundamentals and the information required to develop a disaster recovery plan.

specific requirements

None

estimated completion time

10 minutes

project steps

1. From the standpoint of minimizing interruption to business operations that result in income, what are the three most critical business activities?
2. What types of detailed information would you need about business activities to be able to identify critical systems?
3. Prepare a justification for a formal backup procedure. Include both the activities and process documentation that would be included in a formal backup procedure.

Figure 2-4 Disaster recovery planning

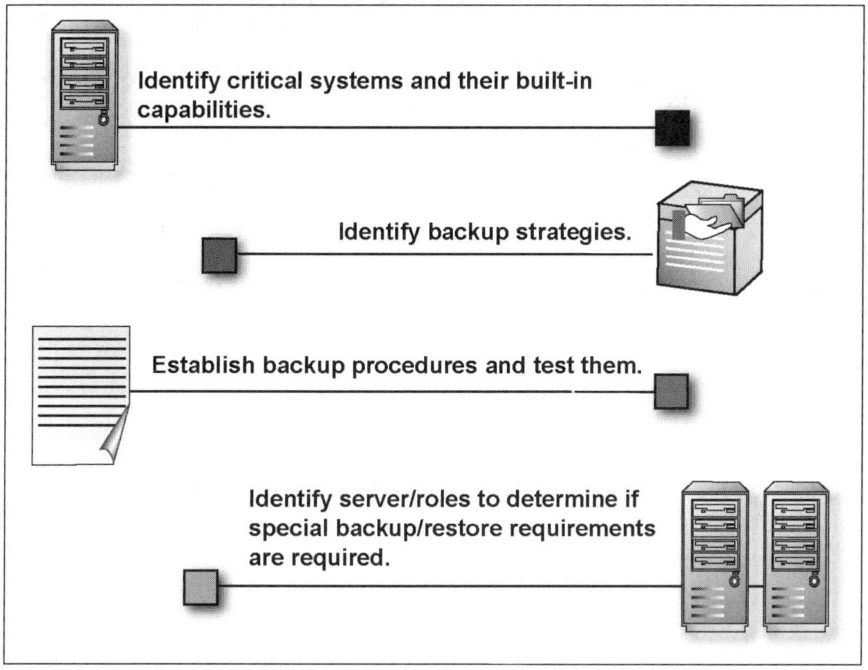

Figure 2-5 Potential disasters

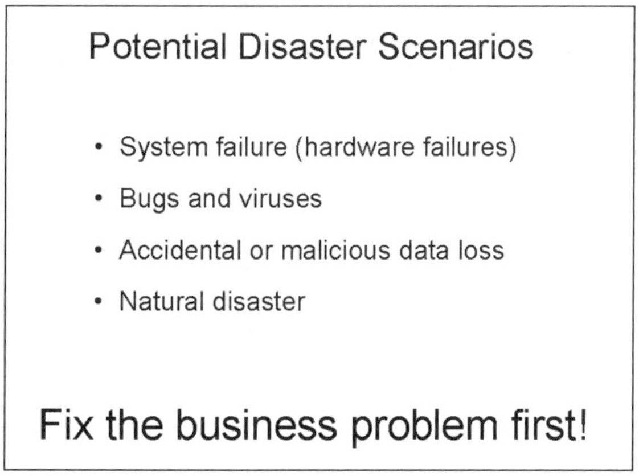

LESSON 3

Analyzing Technical and Interoperability Constraints

Unless you are building a new network from the ground up, any security design must consider legacy systems. Legacy systems include hardware and software which, although not the most up-to-date versions, are often filling mission-critical roles in the business. You must identify the roles filled by legacy systems and the limitations they impose on:

- Hardware
  - Compatibility with chosen technologies
  - Performance
  - Ability to upgrade
- Operating systems
  - Compatibility with network environment
  - Ability to upgrade to more recent versions
  - Available updates (service packs and hot fixes)
- Applications
  - Compatibility with client and server operating systems
  - Special security, user, and environmental requirements
  - Special support hardware requirements

The older the network and the more diverse the network environment, the more likely you are to be faced with legacy systems. Identify legacy systems during the analysis phase. The earlier in the process you address legacy systems; the easier it is to develop an acceptable, cost-effective solution. There are three possible resolutions:

- Remove the legacy system from the network
- Upgrade or patch legacy systems to mitigate security risks
- Leave the system in place and adjust security as necessary

A realistic solution typically includes a mix of these, replacing legacy hardware and software where cost-effective, applying upgrades and fixes where available, and (when no other solution is available) working around the legacy system. The presence of legacy systems also means you need to invest more time and effort testing your security solution to identify potential hidden incompatibilities. Questions you must consider when proposing your specific solution include:

- What security shortcomings does the legacy system introduce?
- Are viable replacements or upgrades available?
- What will it cost to replace the system?
- What will it cost to update or upgrade the system?
- What is the business impact (cost, productivity, etc.) of the solution?

Even the best compromise solution is not without its pitfalls. You might be left with unavoidable weaknesses in your final security design or be unable to implement secure technologies that you want to use. The company could be left owning or locked into a long-term lease for hardware or software that cannot be used in the new network environment.

Scenario

You are working with a team made of up individuals from each of the United States offices to identify security requirements and draft a security plan. It has taken longer than you had hoped to get some of the background information that you need. This situation was not completely unexpected. You have started drafting an ideal security design, describing a proposed security solution, including technologies that you want to introduce.

You finally received a relatively complete network inventory. Most of the server applications are running on either Windows 2000 or Windows Server 2003, but there are a small number of Windows NT servers still in place. Over 70% of the client systems are running Windows 2000 Professional or Windows XP Professional. Most of the remaining systems are running Windows 98 with a small number of Windows 95 clients. You are told that the Windows 95 clients are already scheduled for replacement before you start phasing in the new security design.

Lesson 3 Analyzing Technical and Interoperability Constraints

Project	Exam 70-298 Objective
3.1 Analyzing Capabilities and Interoperability Issues of the Existing Infrastructure	**Analyze technical constraints when designing security.** Identify capabilities of the existing infrastructure. Analyze interoperability constraints.
3.2 Addressing Technology Limitations	**Analyze technical constraints when designing security.** Identify technology limitations.

General Requirements

There are no special requirements for this lesson. However, you may find it helpful to refer to Lesson 3 in your Prentice Hall Certification Series Exam 70-298 textbook for additional information about the topics covered by the projects in this lesson.

project 3.1

Analyzing Capabilities and Interoperability Issues of the Existing Infrastructure

exam objective

Analyze technical constraints when designing security. Identify capabilities of the existing infrastructure. Analyze interoperability constraints.

overview

After receiving the hardware and software inventory for the United States region, you realize that you must adjust your security design. Start by identifying known legacy devices **(Figure 3-1)** and the possible concerns they present. Your initial "wish list" design includes:

- Kerberos-only logon and authentication.
- Encrypt inter-site communication using Internet Protocol Security (IPSec).
- Encrypt finance server access using IPSec (local and remote).
- Manage user and group properties through Group Policy.
- Distribute and update common applications through Group Policy.

Consider options for dealing with legacy systems **(Figure 3-2)**. You must determine the most secure and most cost-effective options. Where there is a difference between the two, you need to have both available for management review.

Learning objective

After completing this project, you will more familiar with the process for identifying legacy devices and have a better understanding of why this is important to security design.

specific requirements

None

estimated completion time

10 minutes

project steps

Identify potential problems with legacy systems in each of the following areas:

1. Kerberos-only authentication.
2. Intra-site use of IPSec.
3. Management through Group Policy.

Figure 3-1 Identifying legacy systems

Legacy Device Concerns

- Hardware
  - BIOS version
  - Network communication speed
  - Hard disk space
  - Available memory
  - Availability of upgrades
- Software
  - Operating system versions
  - Operating system upgrade
  - Server applications
  - Client applications
  - Security requirements
  - Direct hardware access

Figure 3-2 Options for addressing legacy systems

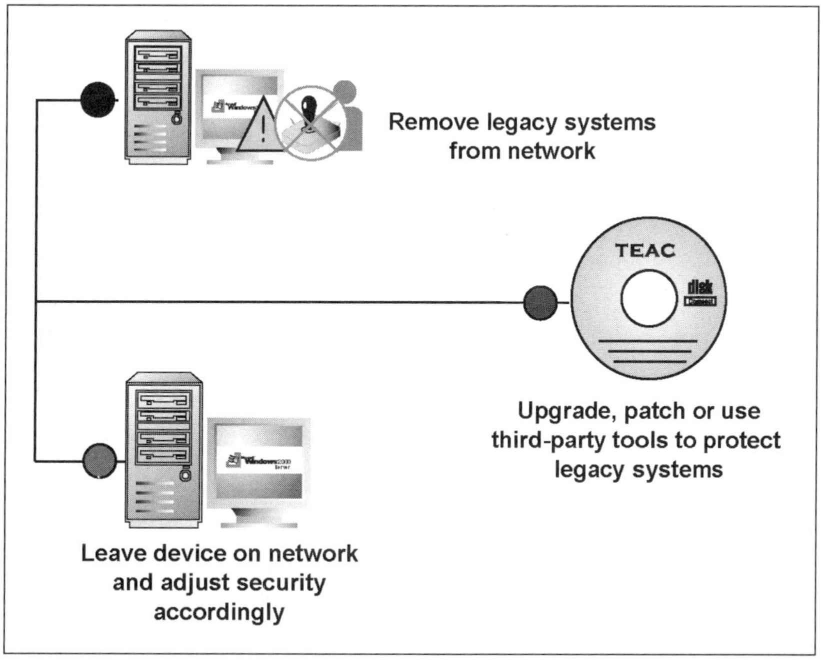

project 3.2 Addressing Technology Limitations

exam objective

Analyze technical constraints when designing security. Identify technology limitations.

overview

Now that you have identified legacy systems present in the network, you must propose plans for addressing the problems they present. Review the network inventory and the shortcomings that you have already identified **(Figure 3-3)**.

learning objective

After completing this project, you will be more familiar with the requirements for addressing legacy systems and other technology limitations.

specific requirements

None

estimated completion time

15 minutes

project steps

1. Based on the preliminary wish list, list the system and application types that will require careful consideration to identify any additional problems you might encounter.
2. Assuming that using IPSec to secure communications with finance servers, what will be required to meet the requirement?
3. Prepare a planning document that identifies problems you might encounter in updating legacy client computers to Windows XP Professional.

The following is an optional hands-on activity. The activity requires access to Windows XP Professional installation files. You will not be installing Windows XP. If your computer is running Windows XP Professional with Service Pack 1 or Service Pack 2 applied, you will not be able to complete the compatibility check.

1. Open a command prompt and navigate to the Windows XP Professional installation files.
2. Start **Setup**.
3. Click **Check system compatibility**.
4. Click **Check my system automatically**.
5. Follow the prompts to check for potential compatibility problems.

Figure 3-3 Inventorying systems on the network

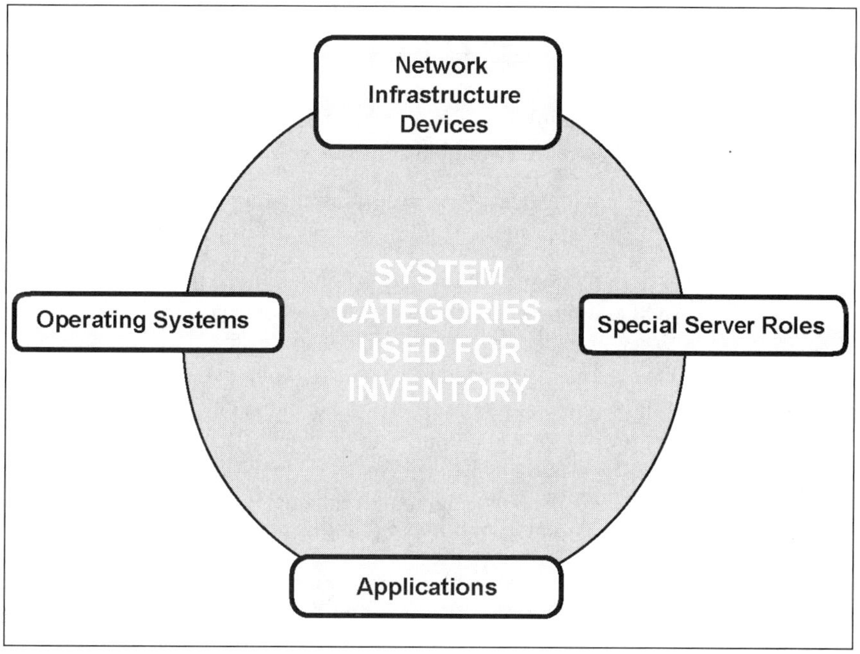

LESSON 4

Designing a Public Key Infrastructure Using Certificate Services

Many security technologies require a Public Key Infrastructure (PKI). A PKI includes one or more Certificate Authorities (CAs), responsible for issuing digital certificates. Digital certificates can be used for a variety of purposes, including:

- Authentication: Includes smart cards, Internet Protocol Security (IPSec), and Secure Sockets Layer (SSL)
- Confidentiality: Includes Encrypting File System (EFS), IPSec, and SSL
- Integrity: Includes digital signatures

For some implementations, purchasing digital certificates from a third-party CA is your best solution. For other implementations, you will want to implement an internal CA hierarchy.

When designing your PKI strategy, you will need to ask a number of questions, including:

- Which users or computers must be issued certificates? For what reasons?
- Where are these users and computers located?
- Do external users need to be able to validate a certificate's authenticity?
- Which operating systems are in use in the environment?
- Who will have the authority to manage certificates and CAs?
- What is the company's certificate revocation policy?
- How will certificates be requested and approved?
- How long will each type of certificate be valid?

The answers to some of these questions will help define the company's Certificate Policy Statement and Certificate Practice Statement. You must create a Certificate Practice Statement for each CA. You also must create a Certificate Policy Statement for each type of certificate issued.

Scenario

You are working with a team made of up individuals from each of the Ready-Biz international offices to identify security requirements and draft a security plan.

You have already completed a network inventory. The current operating systems are summarized below:

- All domain controllers are running Windows Server 2003.
- Most of the server applications are running on either Windows 2000 or Windows Server 2003.
- There are a small number of Windows NT servers still in place.
- Over 70% of the client systems are running Windows 2000 Professional or Windows XP Professional.
- About 25% of the client systems run Windows 98 with a small number of Windows 95 clients. You are told that the Windows 95 clients are already scheduled for replacement before you start phasing in the new security design.

As you revisit the security requirements of your organization, you realize that there are a number of technologies that require digital certificates. These requirements include:

- Encrypt inter-site communication using IPSec.
- Encrypt finance server access using IPSec (remote).
- Secure access to the e-commerce Web site hosted in Chicago.
- Authenticated access for key business partners to an extranet Web site hosted in London.
- EFS encryption for company-confidential data.
- Secure e-mail for internal communication.

Business partner relationships can be long-term, but are more often tied to a specific project.

Now you and the team need to begin designing the Public Key Infrastructure that will support the technologies you plan to implement.

Lesson 4 Designing a Public Key Infrastructure Using Certificate Services

Project	Exam 70-298 Objective
4.1 Understanding Certification Authority Hierarchies	**Design a public key infrastructure (PKI) that uses Certificate Services.** Design a certification authority (CA) hierarchy implementation. Types include geographical, organizational, and trusted.
4.2 Understanding the Enrollment and Distribution Processes	**Design a public key infrastructure (PKI) that uses Certificate Services.** Design enrollment and distribution processes.
4.3 Understanding the Renewal, Revocation, and Auditing Processes	**Design a public key infrastructure (PKI) that uses Certificate Services.** Establish renewal, revocation, and auditing processes.
4.4 Securing Certification Authority Servers	**Design a public key infrastructure (PKI) that uses Certificate Services.** Designing security for CA servers.

General Requirements

There are no special requirements for this lesson. However, you may find it helpful to refer to Lesson 4 in your Prentice Hall Certification Series Exam 70-298 textbook for additional information about the topics covered by the projects in this lesson.

project 4.1

Understanding Certification Authority Hierarchies

exam objective

Design a public key infrastructure (PKI) that uses Certificate Services. Design a certification authority (CA) hierarchy implementation. Types include geographical, organizational, and trusted.

overview

You must determine the most secure and most cost-effective hierarchy for issuing certificates. You will consider geographical and organizational requirements.

Refer to **Table 4-1** for a review of each type of CA.

Learning objective

After completing this project, you will understand how to design a CA hierarchy to meet geographical and organizational requirements.

specific requirements

None

estimated completion time

15 minutes

project steps

1. Prepare a PowerPoint or other form of presentation that illustrates the proposed hierarchy. Identify each CA as a standalone or enterprise CA. Give justification for your design by discussing how it meets the following objectives:
   - Each international region must be autonomous.
   - User and computer certificates must be distributed in each local office.
   - CA certificates must be issued automatically from a regional server.
   - Autoenrollment is supported.
   - The root CA or CAs must be secured from compromise.
2. Which certificate or certificates should be issued by the internal hierarchy? Which are best issued by a third-party CA?

Table 4-1 Certification Authority characteristics

Enterprise root CA	• Requires that Active Directory be available. • Certificate requests can be made by using Certification Request Wizard or via Web Support pages. • Uses information in Active Directory to verify the security principal's identity. • Installed on a Windows Server 2003/Windows 2000 server that is a member of an Active Directory domain.
Standalone root CA	• Does not require Active Directory to function. • Certificate requests can be made by using Web Support pages. • More information from the requester of the certificate is required if Active Directory is not used. • Can be a member of an Active Directory domain but not required. • Installed on a Windows Server 2003/Windows 2000 Server that is or is not a member of an Active Directory domain.
Subordinate enterprise CA	• Requires that Active Directory be available. • Certificate requests can be made by using Certification Request Wizard or via Web Support pages. • Uses information in Active Directory to verify the security principal's identity. • Installed on a Windows Server 2003/Windows 2000 Server that is a member of an Active Directory domain.
Subordinate standalone CA	• Does not require Active Directory to function. • Certificate requests can be made by using Web Support pages. • More information from the requester of the certificate is required if Active Directory is not used. • Receives its certificate from a root CA. • Installed on a Windows Server 2003/Windows 2000 Server that is or is not a member of an Active Directory domain.

project 4.2

Understanding the Enrollment and Distribution Processes

exam objective

Design a public key infrastructure (PKI) that uses Certificate Services. Design enrollment and distribution processes.

overview

Now that you designed the hierarchy, you must determine how certificates will be enrolled and distributed. You will consider which certificates will be enrolled using autoenrollment and which will be requested using the Web Enrollment Support Pages **(Figure 4-1)**.

You will also determine which certificates will be automatically approved and which require manual verification and approval. The factors you will consider are listed in **Table 4-2**.

learning objective

After completing this project, you will understand the factors you must consider when designing a certificate enrollment and distribution strategy.

specific requirements

None

estimated completion time

10 minutes

project steps

1. Create a table that describes the certificates, who they must be distributed to, and the enrollment method that will be used. Consider the following:
   - Client operating system requirements
   - Automatic or manual approval
2. What operating system must you install Certificate Services on to support automatic enrollment of secure e-mail certificates?
3. Which certificates will require manual approval?
4. What Windows component must be installed to support Web Support Enrollment Pages?
5. Which certificate requires a short validity period?

Figure 4-1 Web Enrollment Support Pages

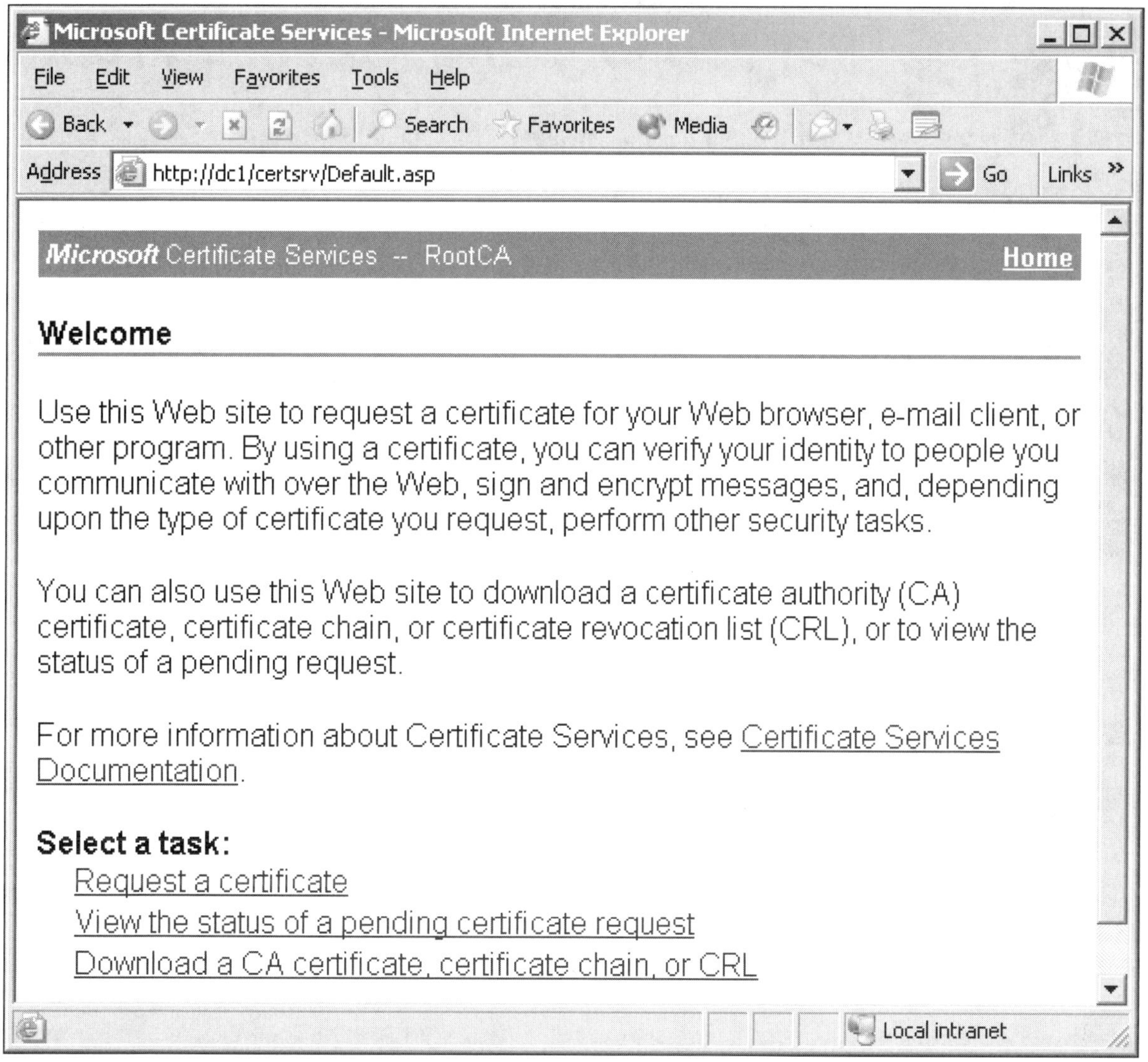

Table 4-2 Factors to be considered in designing the certificate enrollment and distribution process

Factor	Related considerations
Operating systems to be used	Are operating systems capable of integrating with Active Directory? Can Certificate Request Wizard be used or will certificates have to be requested using Web Enrollment Support pages?
Type of CA that will issue certificates	Enterprise CA required for smart card enrollment stations. Enterprise CA required for auto enrollment of certificates.
Validity period of certificates	If certificates are to be used for a short-term project, may need to shorten default validity period.
Approval process to be used	If a large number of certificates must be distributed, it's better to use automatic enrollment. If using sensitive certificates that allow a wide range of privileges, use manual enrollment.

project 4.3

Understanding the Renewal, Revocation, and Auditing Processes

exam objective

Design a public key infrastructure (PKI) that uses Certificate Services. Establish renewal, revocation, and auditing processes.

overview

Now that you have determined how certificates will be enrolled and distributed, you need to design a strategy for revoking certificates, publishing the Certificate Revocation List (CRL), and renewing certificates.

Renewal can occur either manually or automatically. You will usually select automatic renewal when automatic enrollment is enabled and in certain cases where manual enrollment is used, but the relationship will continue past the lifetime of the certificate. You will use manual enrollment when you want to be able to reevaluate the certificate's validity periodically. You must consider four key factors when designing a certificate revocation strategy:

- Under what circumstances should a certificate be revoked?
- Who makes the decision to revoke a certificate?
- Where should the CRL be published?
- Can delta CRLs be used?

The revocation process is summarized in **Figure 4-2**.

learning objective

After completing this project, you will understand the factors you must consider when designing a certificate renewal and revocation policy.

specific requirements

You must have completed Projects 4.1 and 4.2.

estimated completion time

15 minutes

project steps

1. Modify the table you created in Project 4.2 to indicate each type of certificate should be renewed.
2. Modify the presentation you created in Project 4.1 to indicate where the CRL for each CA will be published. Consider the following requirements:
   - Does the server issue certificates that must be validated by external users?
   - Is the CA offline or online?
3. Identify the operating systems that must be upgraded before delta CRLs can be used effectively.

Figure 4-2 Revocation processes

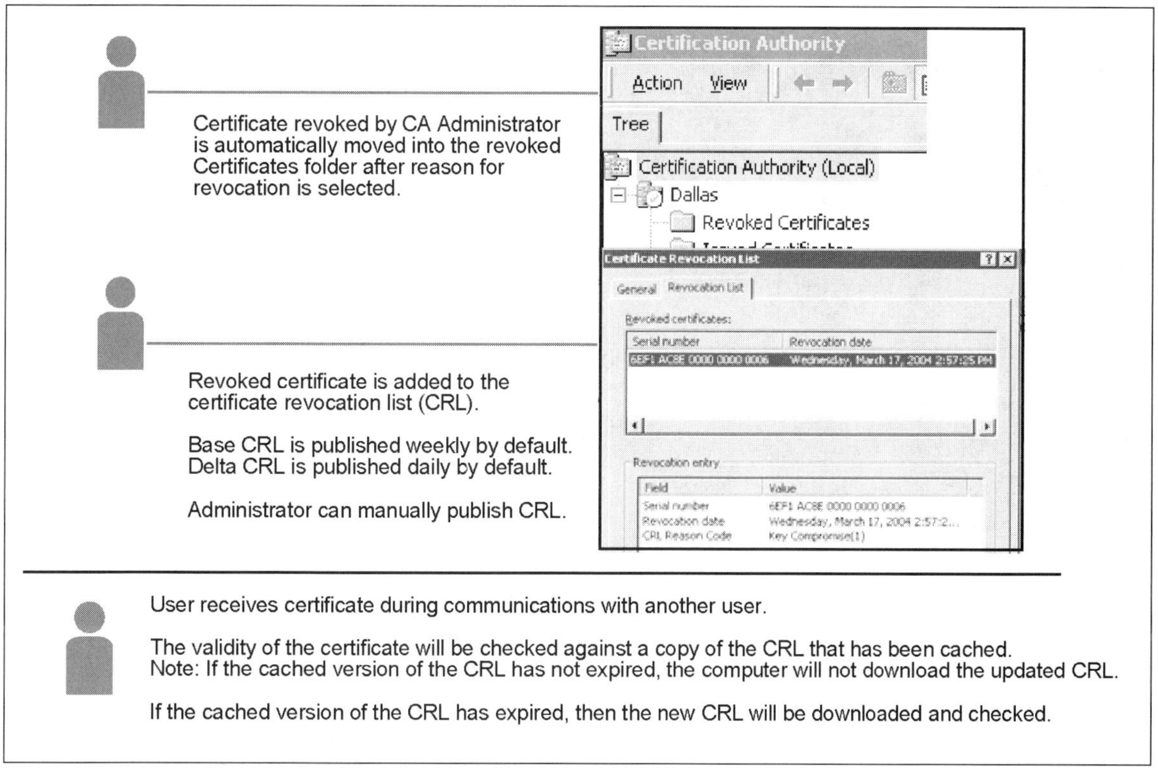

project 4.4

Securing Certification Authority Servers

exam objective

Design a public key infrastructure (PKI) that uses Certificate Services. Designing security for CA servers.

overview

Now that you have designed a Public Key Infrastructure, you must assess whether it is as secure as it can be. Some potential vulnerabilities are illustrated in **Figure 4-3**.

Your first step in assessing your PKI is to identify the potential security threats. Next, you must take steps to mitigate the threats. A few steps you can take are shown in **Figure 4-4**.

learning objective

After completing this project, you will be able to identify threats to a PKI and steps that can be taken to mitigate those threats.

specific requirements

You must have completed Projects 4.1, 4.2, and 4.3.

estimated completion time

10 minutes

project steps

1. Evaluate the hierarchy you proposed in Projects 4-1 and 4-3. Answer the following questions?
   - Are the root CAs sufficiently protected against attack?
   - Are there CRLs that represent a single point of failure?
2. Evaluate the certificate enrollment, distribution, and renewal strategy you proposed in Projects 4-1 and 4-2. Which permissions must be granted to permit autoenrollment?

Figure 4-3 Possible attacks against certification authorities

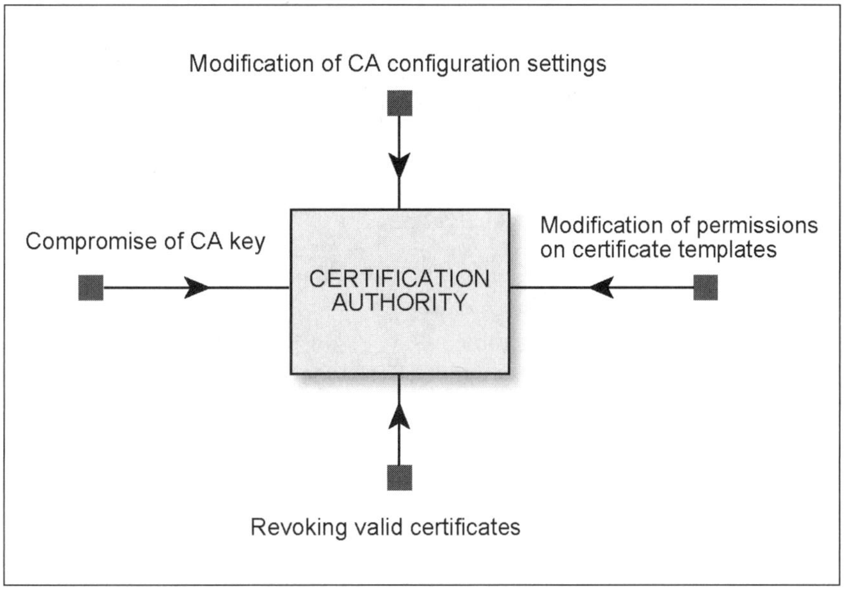

Figure 4-4 Design considerations for a secure CA

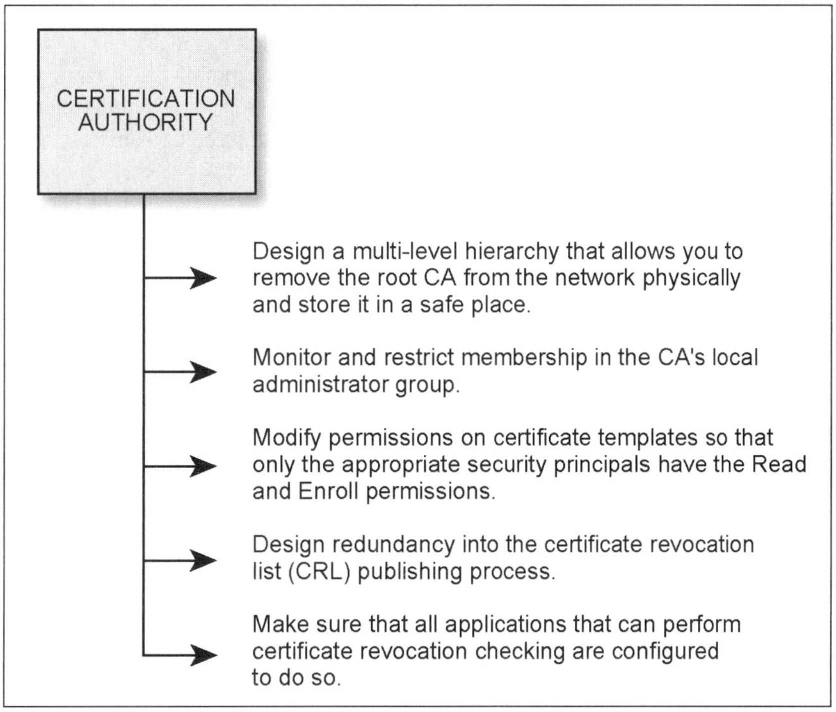

LESSON 5

Designing Security for Network Management

Security problems can result from a number of different causes. Sometimes, the security design itself is at fault. However, often a security problem may be created as a result of the failure of those responsible for implementing and maintaining the security design to do so properly. For instance, security problems can be introduced if:

- Network administrators are improperly or incompletely trained.
- Network administrators do not understand components of the security design or their justification.
- Temporary changes are made as a convenience and never corrected.
- Administrative rights are delegated at inappropriate levels or to inappropriate users.

It is important to understand these potential shortcomings and consider them in your security design. Analysis of the tasks performed by network administrators, and how they are performed, can be a critical part of the analysis phase and can directly impact how a security design is implemented.

Security design should be based on the principle of least privilege, that users should be given no more privileges than necessary to perform their job functions. Two key elements of understanding how this is implemented in your design are:

- Autonomy—Independent management of resources by administrators, overridden by higher administrative authority, if necessary (non-exclusive control).
- Isolation—Independent management of resources by administrators without the ability of other administrators to take over resources (exclusive control).

Your domain design will depend on whether your ultimate goal is autonomy, isolation, or some mix of the two. In your design, the Active Directory forest is your security boundary, providing a way to isolate administration through a multiple forest design. The Active Directory domain is your security policy boundary, implementing separate security policies but implementing autonomy through the overriding control of administrators in a parent domain.

Within your design, administrators must know the tools available and understand their proper use. These include:

- Microsoft Management Console (MMC)—Shell hosting administrative tool snap-ins with the ability to create custom management tools sets targeted to management requirements.
- Terminal Server—Provides for remote server (and domain controller) administrator through Remote Desktop for Administration (RDA).
- Telnet—Supports remote logon and remote execution of command-line utilities.

Emergency Management Services (EMS) was introduced with Windows Server 2003. The relative newness of this feature might result in its security being overlooked. You must consider how EMS is implemented and whether you are relying on in-band (standard connections an administrator would use to connect to another computer over the network or via its local console) or out-of-band connections (management of a server by using a special port or device, such as a terminal concentrator or service processor).

Depending on your situation, out-of-band connections require you to consider interface options, including:

- **Console redirection:** Enabled at computer to allow transmission of text data through management port.
- **Service processors:** Provide interface as Telnet console or Web browser and are implemented through an adapter card or server circuitry.
- **Terminal concentrations:** Single network interface for viewing multiple servers.

When considering out-of-band management interfaces, you must include the security mechanisms supported and include physical access security in your design.

Scenario

You are continuing to work with Ready-Biz in designing security for the United States division. Even though the plan is to duplicate applicable parts of the plan designed for the United States across each division, each international division will remain responsible for its own administration.

Lesson 5 Designing Security for Network Management

Project	Exam 70-298 Objective
5.1 Managing the Risk of Managing Networks	**Design security for network management**. Manage the risk of managing networks.
5.2 Designing the Administration of Servers Using Common Tools	**Design security for network management**. Design the administration by of servers by using common administration tools. Tools include Microsoft Management Console (MMC), Terminal Server, Remote Desktop for Administration, Remote Assistance, and Telnet.
5.3 Securing Emergency Management Services	**Design security for network management**. Design security for Emergency Management Services.

General Requirements

There are no special requirements for this lesson. However, you may find it helpful to refer to Lesson 5 in your Prentice Hall Certification Series Exam 70-298 textbook for additional information about the topics covered by the projects in this lesson.

project 5.1

Managing the Risk of Managing Networks

exam objective

Design security for network management. Manage the risk of managing networks.

overview

You must review the interim network design and the established domain model, specifically considering the principle of least privilege **(Figure 5-1)**. You must determine if the Active Directory design is compatible with the security design and what, if any, change must be made. Key considerations include:

- Each division is managed as a separate entity.
- Regional offices are under ultimate control of the main divisional office.

A representation of the current Active Directory design is shown in **Figure 5-2**. No cross-forest trusts have been established. The child domains represent the regional offices, but not all regional offices are shown, for the sake of simplicity.

learning objective

After completing this project, you will be more familiar with the relationship between implementing autonomy and isolation in a security design and Active Directory design models.

specific requirements

None

estimated completion time

15 minutes

project steps

1. Prepare a brief report describing how well the Active Directory design matches the autonomy and isolation requirements in the security design. Be specific in your description.
2. List management areas that will be the same through a division and what management areas that can be controlled at the regional offices.

Figure 5-1 Principle of least privilege

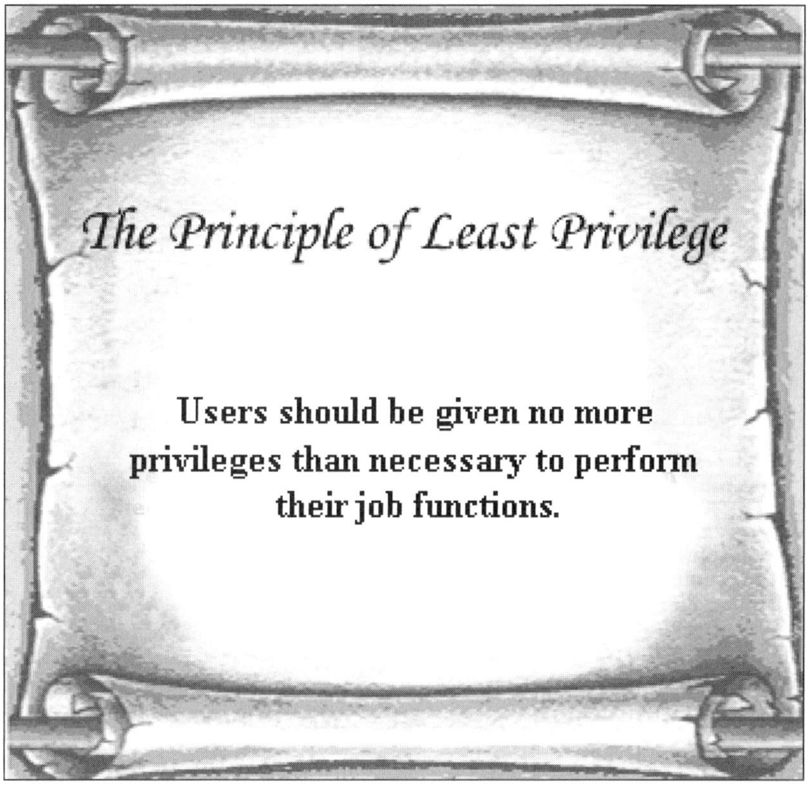

Figure 5-2 Ready-Biz Active Directory domain design

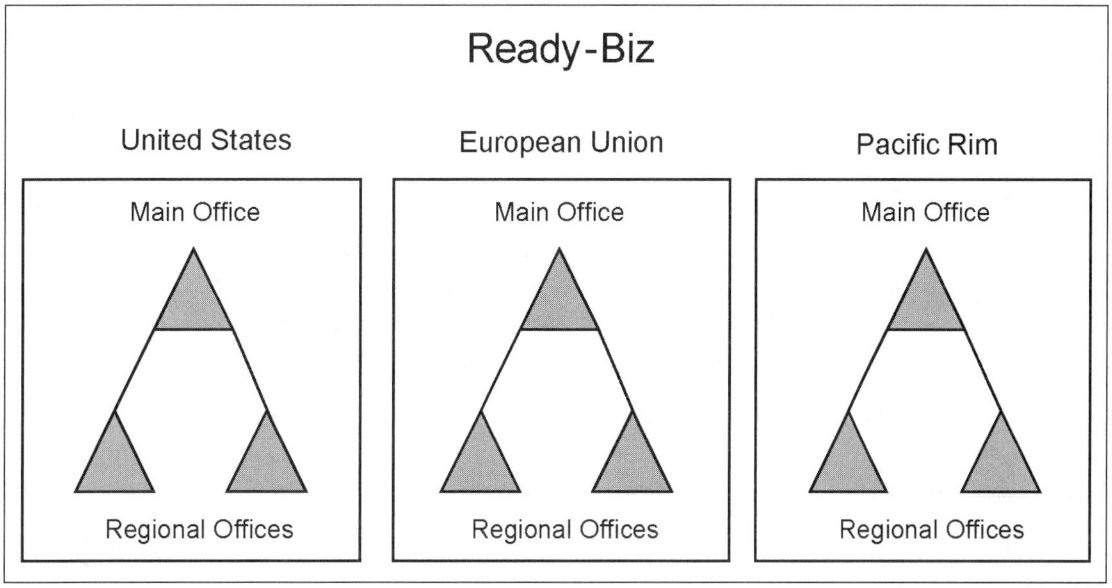

project 5.2

Designing Administration of Services by Using Common Tools

exam objective

Design security for network management. Design the administration of servers by using common administration tools. Tools include Microsoft Management Console (MMC), Terminal Server, Remote Desktop for Administration, Remote Assistance, and Telnet.

overview

Based on your recommendation, a new security department is established in the Chicago office as a separate entity from the information technology (IT) department. Candidates for regional security department personnel are now in progress. The number of full administrators will be strictly limited with several users delegated to specific management tasks. The current identified tasks are:

- Domain Name System (DNS) management (Chicago only)
- Dynamic Host Configuration Protocol (DHCP) management (each office)
- User and group account management (each office, by department)
- Logon and password control (each office)

Full administrators in the Chicago office will be able to override management decisions made in any regional office.

You are working with the security department to determine which tools **(Figure 5-3)** are best matched to each security task.

learning objective

After completing this project, you will be able to identify the best security tools to use for specific administrative tasks and management situations.

specific requirements

None

estimated completion time

15 minutes

project steps

1. How can the MMC be used to implement the principle of least privilege for delegated administrative tasks?
2. What specific custom management consoles are needed to meet the identified administrative requirements?
3. You want to ensure that the highest possible level of security is used when directly administering domain controllers from a remote location. Describe how you can use Terminal Services to meet this requirement **(Figure 5-4** and **Figure 5-5**).

Figure 5-3 Available management tools

- Microsoft Management Console (MMC)
  - Custom Management Consoles
  - Control Over Management Tools
- Terminal Services
  - Remote Desktop for Administration (RDA)
  - Remote Assistance
- Telnet

Figure 5-4 Enabling Remote Desktop Administration

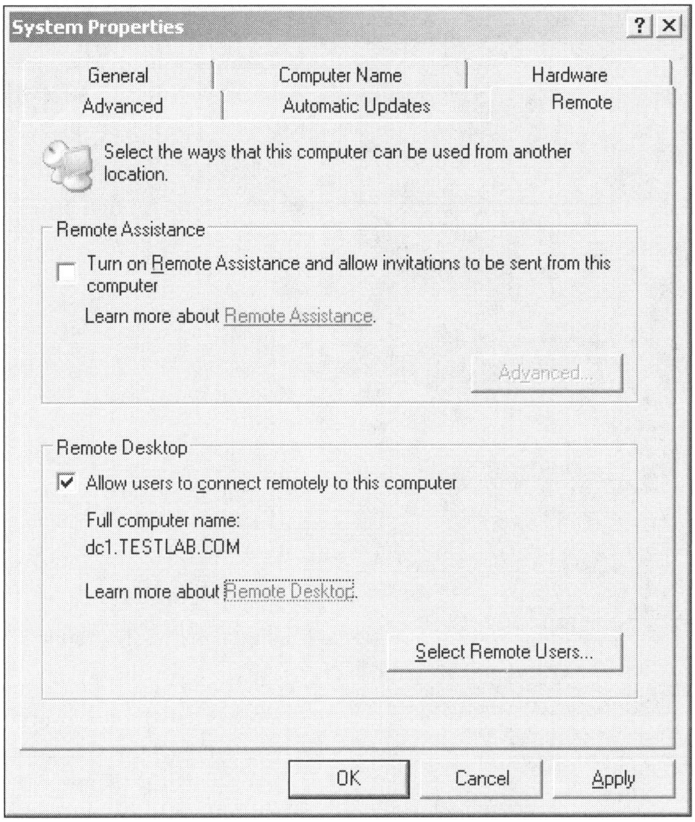

Figure 5-5 Terminal Services encryption settings

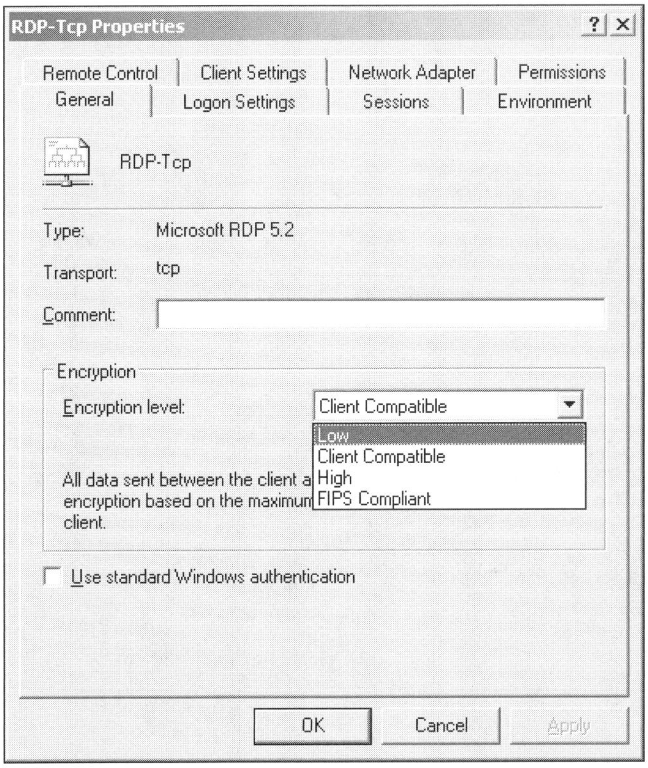

project 5.3

Securing Emergency Management Services

exam objective

Design security for network management. Design security for Emergency Management Services.

overview

A recently added requirement to the security design is a need to secure Emergency Management Services (EMS). You must compare communication options **(Figure 5-6)** to determine the best solution.

learning objective

After completing this project, you will understand EMS communication options and their security requirements.

specific requirements

None

estimated completion time

15 minutes

project steps

Prepare a memo that reports your findings on the following topics:

1. What are the in-band and out-of-band communication options available?
2. What are the hardware requirements if you want to use a terminal concentrator for communications with all domain controllers in each office **(Figure 5-7)**?
3. What are the requirements for using Telnet with servers in remote offices?
4. How can Telnet traffic be secured?

Figure 5-6 Examples of in-band and out-of-band communications

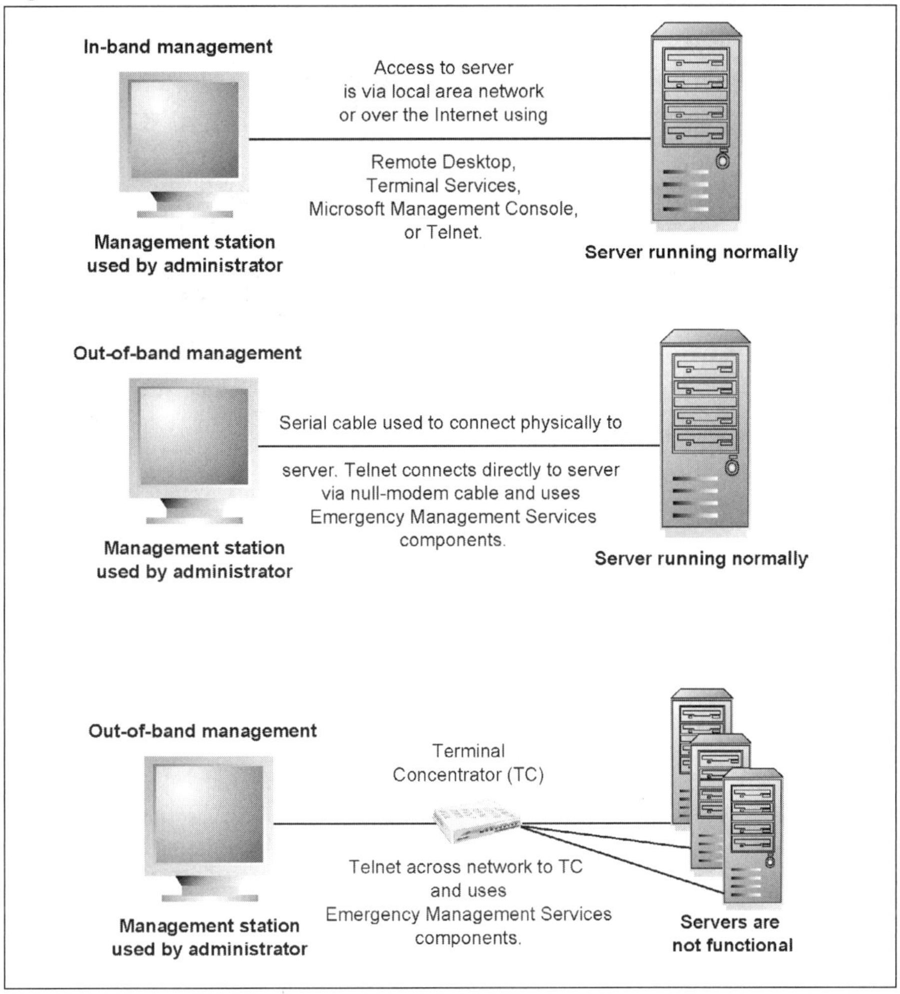

Figure 5-7 Example of terminal concentrator

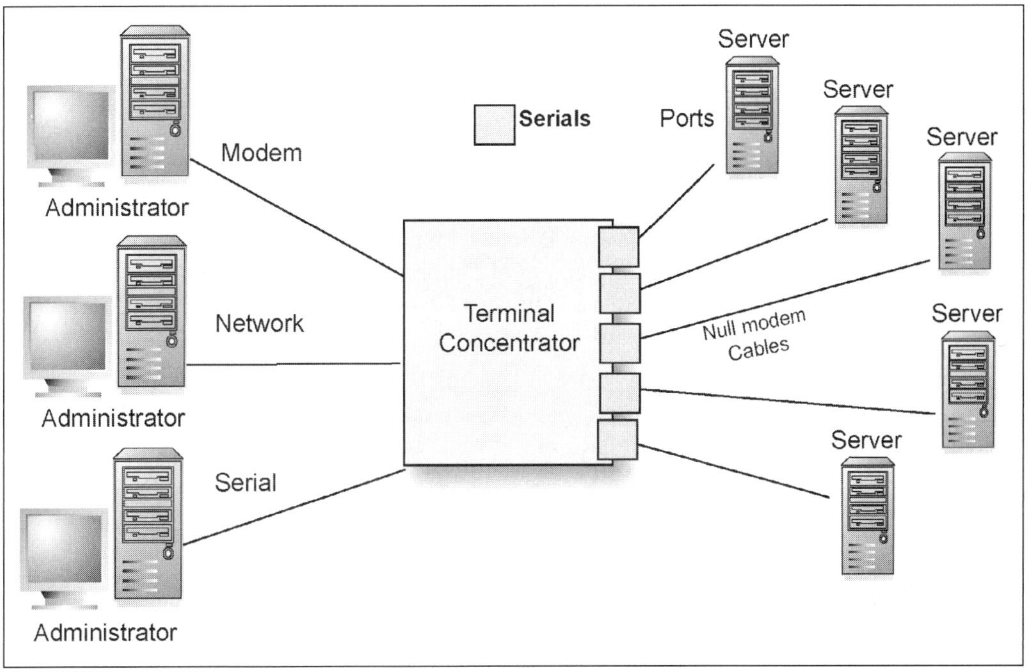

LESSON

6 Designing a Security Update Infrastructure

Protecting your network against threats requires constant diligence. Potential attackers are constantly searching for new ways to exploit the operating system. When a new type of attack is launched, Microsoft works to create a security patch to resolve the problem. It is the responsibility of network administrators to ensure that security patches are tested and deployed in a timely manner.

Fortunately, several tools are available to help administrators evaluate systems to determine their patch level and deploy patches to the computers to which they should be applied. Some of these include:

- Windows Update and Automatic Updates
- Software Update Services (SUS)
- Group Policy
- Systems Management Server (SMS)
- Microsoft Baseline Security Analyzer (MBSA)

Part of your job when designing a security infrastructure is to determine when and how each of these tools should be used. The focus in this lesson is on SUS, Group Policy, and MBSA.

A SUS server is used to manage the approval and deployment of updates internally. The SUS server downloads updates from the Microsoft Windows Update Web site. A network administrator can then test those updates and approve the ones that are appropriate for the SUS clients.

Group Policy can be used to configure clients to use a specific SUS server and to prevent users from updating their computers manually using Windows Update. Policies related to updates are located under Computer Configuration, Administrative Templates, Windows Components, Windows Update.

MBSA is a tool you can download from Microsoft's Web site. It is used to scan a computer for its update status and well-known vulnerabilities caused by non-secure configuration settings. It checks the configuration of the operating system, IIS 4.0 and later, SQL Server, Internet Explorer 5.01 and later, Office 2000, and Office XP.

Scenario

You are working with a team made up of individuals from each of the Ready-Biz offices in the United States to develop an update infrastructure. The United States plan will be used as a model in the international offices.

You have already completed a network inventory. The current operating systems are summarized below:

- All domain controllers are running Windows Server 2003.
- Most of the server applications are running on either Windows 2000 or Windows Server 2003.
- There are a small number of Windows NT servers still in place.
- Over 70% of the client systems are running Windows 2000 Professional or Windows XP Professional.
- About 25% of the client systems run Windows 98 with a small number of Windows 95 clients. You are told that the Windows 95 clients are already scheduled for replacement before you start phasing in the new security design.

The computers in the manufacturing facility run proprietary applications. Past experience has shown that these applications are likely to have compatibility issues with some types of security patches. Still, you want to ensure that these computers are patched with all compatible patches. The other computers in the organization need to be kept as up-to-date as possible. However, all patches should be tested in the Chicago office before they are deployed to client computers.

Lesson 6 Designing a Security Update Infrastructure

Project	*Exam 70-298 Objective*
6.1 Designing a Software Update Services Infrastructure	**Design a security update infrastructure**. Design a Software Update Services (SUS) infrastructure.
6.2 Using Group Policy to Deploy Software Updates	**Design a security update infrastructure**. Design Group Policy to deploy software updates.
6.3 Designing Strategies for Identifying and Patching Computers	**Design a security update infrastructure.** Design a strategy for identifying computers that are not at the current patch level.

General Requirements

In order to complete Project 6.3, you will need administrative rights on a computer that supports MBSA (Windows 2000, Windows XP Professional, or Windows Server 2003) and that can access the Internet. You may also find it helpful to refer to Lesson 6 in your Prentice Hall Certification Series Exam 70-298 textbook for additional information about the topics covered by the projects in this lesson.

project 6.1

Designing a Software Update Services Infrastructure

exam objective

Design a security update infrastructure. Design a Software Update Services (SUS) infrastructure.

overview

You must design the best infrastructure for deploying security updates and service packs. You will consider geographical, organizational, and application requirements.

You must provide documentation to support the use of SUS servers to deploy updates. You must also design a SUS hierarchy to meet your requirements.

As you'll recall, SUS can be implemented with a single parent SUS server **(Figure 6-1)** or you can implement a separate parent SUS server for the test lab **(Figure 6-2)**.

learning objective

After completing this project, you will more familiar with designing a SUS hierarchy to meet organizational, application compatibility, and geographical requirements.

specific requirements

None

estimated completion time

20 minutes

project steps

1. Prepare a PowerPoint or other form of presentation that outlines the benefits of using SUS to deploy updates and service packs.
2. Add a diagram of the proposed SUS hierarchy to your presentation. Make sure to consider the following requirements:
   - Computers in the manufacturing department will not support all updates.
   - All updates will be tested and approved in Chicago.
   - Clients should contact a SUS server in their local office.
3. There has been talk about isolating certain computers from the Internet. How will this change the design?

Figure 6-1 A single parent-child SUS hierarchy

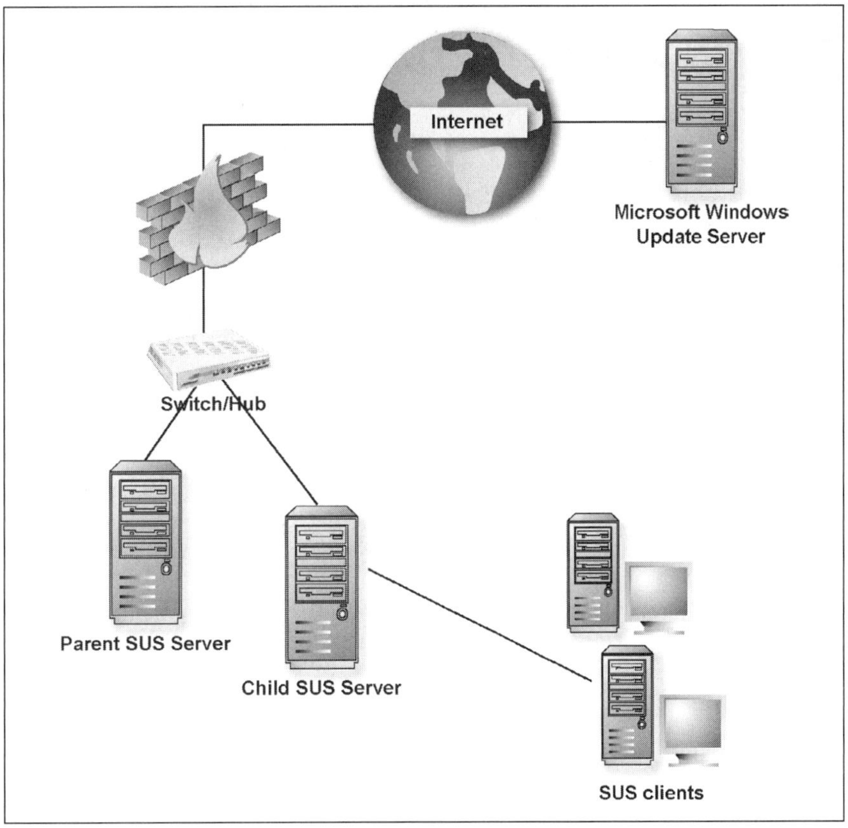

Figure 6-2 Separate SUS hierarchies

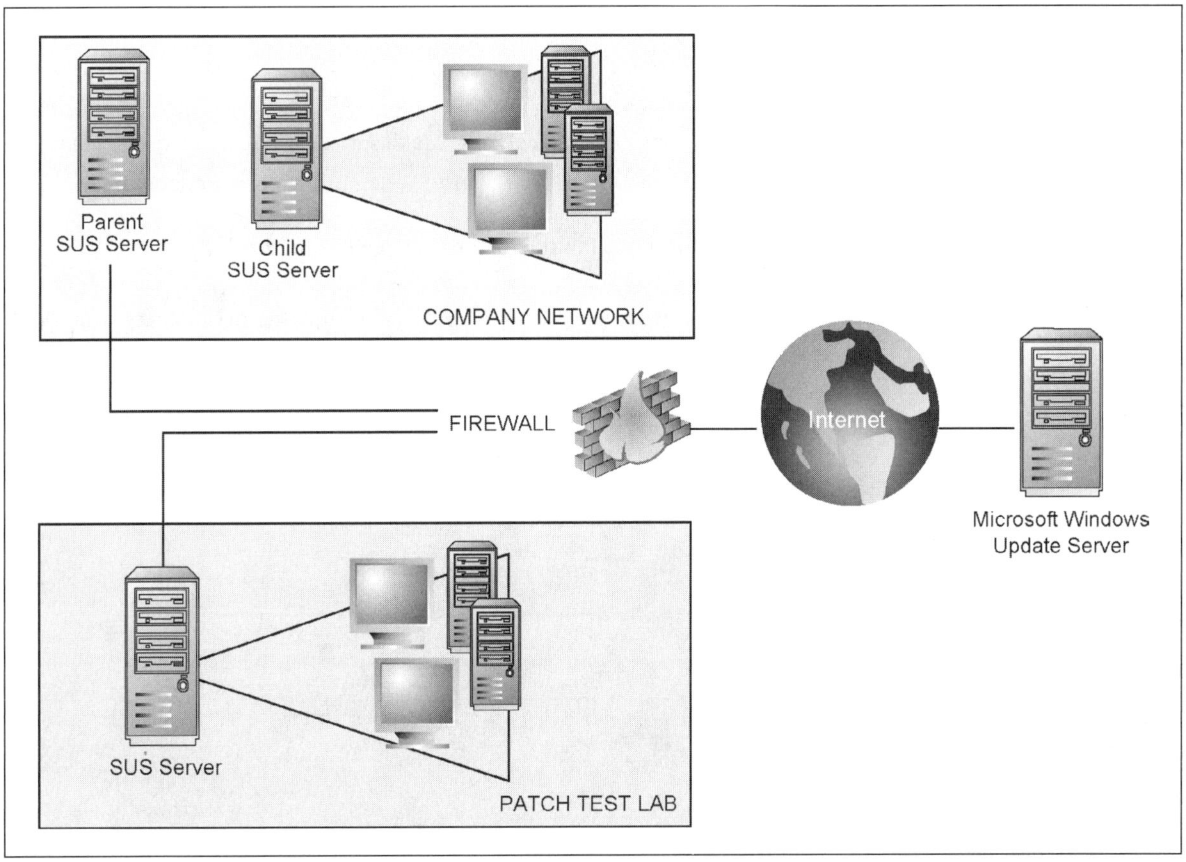

project 6.2

Using Group Policy to Deploy Software Updates

exam objective

Design a security update infrastructure. Design Group Policy to deploy software updates.

overview

Now that you designed the hierarchy, you must determine how clients will be configured to access the SUS servers. You must create a presentation that outlines the benefits for configuring client computers using Group Policy. As you'll recall, the Ready-Biz Active Directory is structured with a root domain in the Chicago office and regional child domains (**Figure 6-3**).

The presentation must also describe where in the hierarchy each GPO will be linked. Each domain is structured with the organizational unit (OU) hierarchy shown in **Figure 6-4**.

Each regional office is its own site. Chicago is also its own site. A domain controller for each regional domain is located at the Chicago site.

learning objective

After completing this project, you will be more familiar with designing a strategy for configuring SUS clients using Group Policy.

specific requirements

None

estimated completion time

10 minutes

project steps

1. Create a PowerPoint or other form of presentation that demonstrates how Group Policy can be used to configure SUS clients. Make sure to consider the following points:
   - People who travel to different offices must download updates from the local SUS server.
   - Computers in the Manufacturing department require different updates from other computers.
2. How can you prevent users from manually updating their computers from the Microsoft Windows Update site?

Figure 6-3 Active Directory design

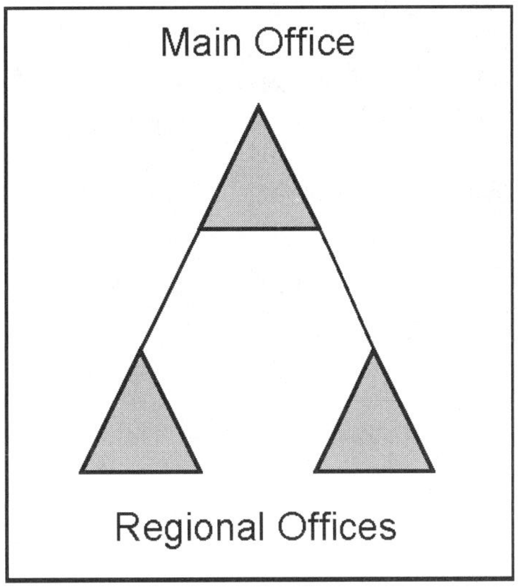

Figure 6-4 Organizational unit hierarchy

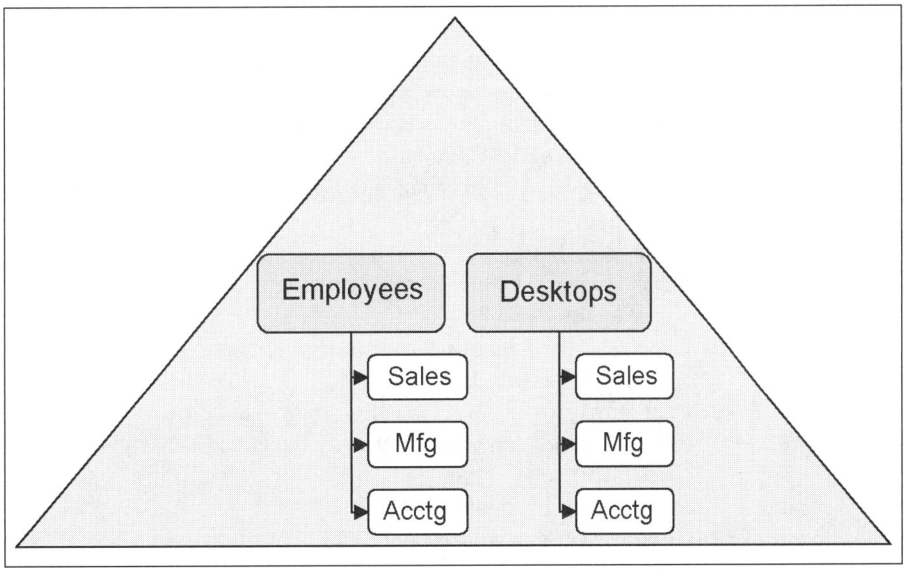

project 6.3

Designing Strategies for Identifying and Patching Computers

exam objective

Design a security update infrastructure. Design a strategy for identifying computers that are not at the current patch level.

overview

Even with an automatic update infrastructure in place, you will want to audit systems to ensure that they have been updated. You need to demonstrate how Microsoft Baseline Security Analyzer (MBSA) can be used to scan systems for missing patches (**Figure 6-5**) and security vulnerabilities (**Figure 6-6**).

learning objective

After completing this project, you will know how to use MBSA to scan a computer. You will also be more familiar with options for scanning multiple computers.

specific requirements

See General Requirements.

estimated completion time

15 minutes

project steps

1. Launch **Internet Explorer** and navigate to the following Web address: **www.microsoft.com/technet/security/tools/mbsahome.mspx**.
2. Click the **Download Now** link.
3. A **File Download - Security Warning** message box will appear, asking if you want to run or save the file. Click **Run**.
4. Depending on the computer's configuration, you may also receive an additional security warning, asking if you want to run this software. Click **Run**.
5. The **MBSA Setup** dialog box appears. Click **Next**.
6. Select the **I accept the license agreement** option button and click **Next**.
7. Next you must choose a destination folder. Accept the default by clicking **Next**.
8. Click **Install** on the **Start Installation** screen.
9. After **MBSA** is installed, click **OK**.
10. Launch **Microsoft Baseline Security Analyzer**. To do so, click **Start**, point to **All Programs** and then click **Microsoft Baseline Security Analyzer**.
11. Click **Scan more than one computer**. What options are available for selecting the computers to be scanned?
12. Click **Pick a computer to scan**. Verify that your computer is listed under **Computer Name**. What options are available for scanning?
13. Click **Start Scan**.
14. Take some time to review the results.
15. Close Microsoft Baseline Security Analyzer.

Figure 6-5 MBSA missing patches report

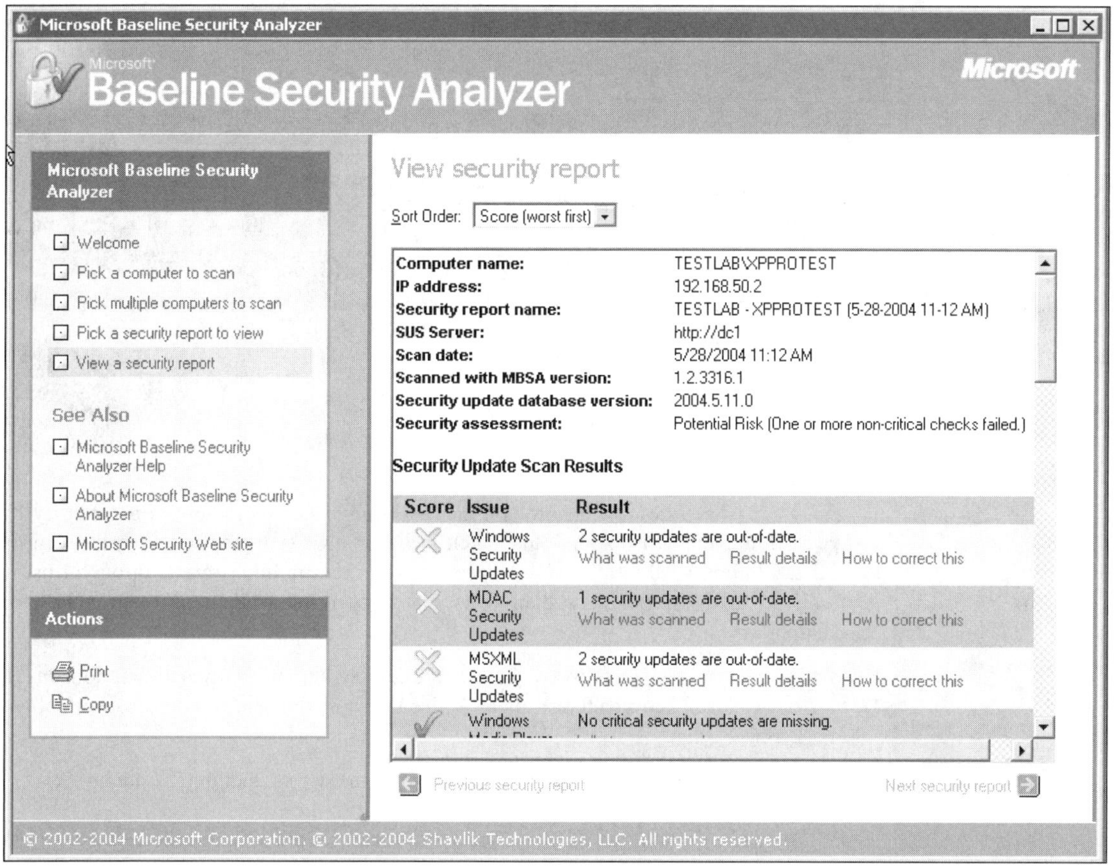

Figure 6-6 MBSA common security vulnerabilities report

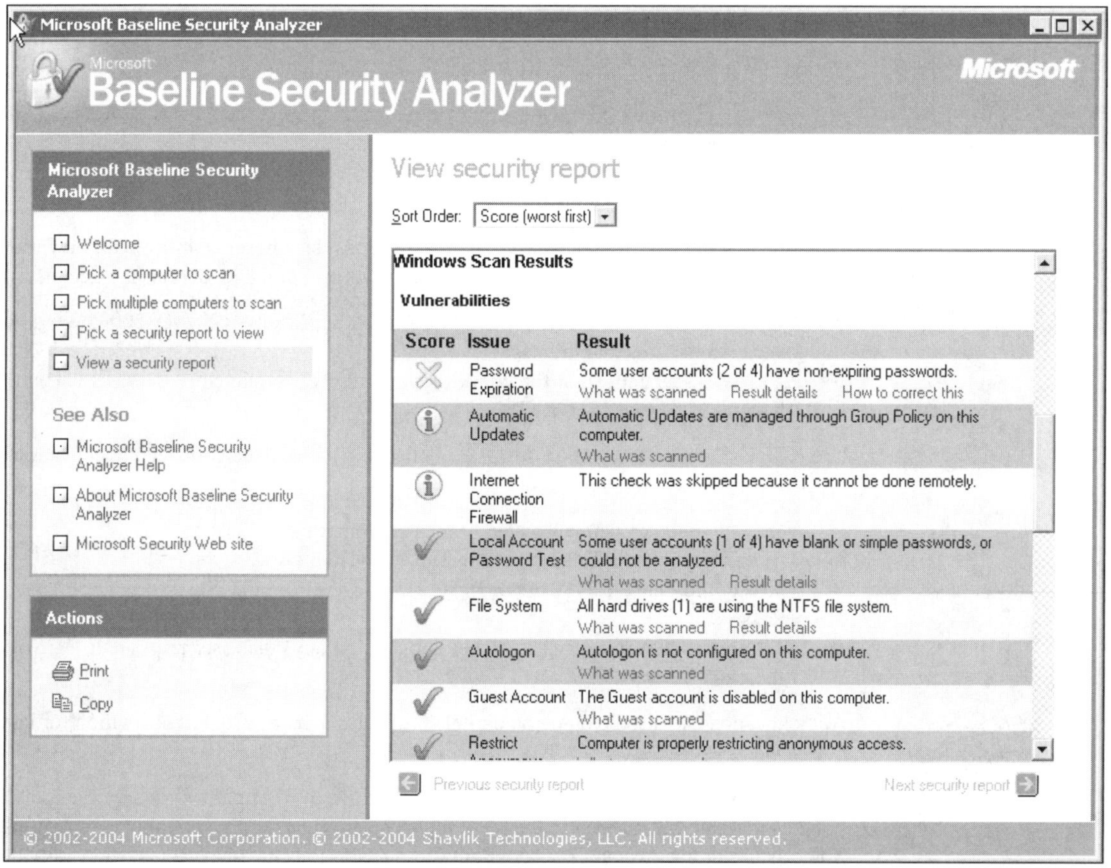

LESSON 7

Designing a Logical Authentication Strategy

Lesson 5 described how you can use Active Directory forests as security boundaries to implement isolation. This is not, however, always appropriate for your security needs. You might need to allow users access to resources in other forests through trust relationships. Designing a security solution that meets your networking needs requires an understanding of trust relationships.

Within a forest, transitive two-way trusts are created automatically between domains. No trusts are created by default between forests. In an Active Directory domain, you can create one-way external trust relationships:

- **Between forests (Forest trust)**: Transitive trust that requires Windows Server 2003 forest functional level.
- **Between domains in different forests (Shortcut trust)**: Non-transitive trust with authentication without following the entire trust path.
- **With Windows NT 4 domains (Shortcut trust)**: Non-transitive trust.

Trusts can be also created with Kerberos realms (such as Unix realms) as one-way or two-way trusts and as transitive or non-transitive trusts.

Options for maximizing security when establishing trusts include:

- **Security identifier (SID) filtering**: Compares the SIDs in the request with the SID of the domain hosting the account. Typically used in security design.
- **Selective authentication**: Explicitly defines domain controllers to which external users can authenticate. Used in limited situations only.

When deploying your security design, you must consider interoperability with down-level and non-Windows clients. Use the strongest authentication protocol possible; options include the following:

- **Kerberos v5**: Authentication for Windows 2000, Windows Server 2003, Windows XP, Unix, Linux, AS400, and mainframes.
- **NTLMv2**: Authentication for Windows 9x (with Active Directory Services Client software) and Windows NT 4 (with Service Pack 4).

Use NTLMv2 only if supporting down-level clients. Kerberos, the stronger authentication, is preferred. Kerberos provides access by:

- Verifying logon credentials by the Authentication Service (AS).
- The user is granted a Ticket Granting Ticket (TGT) by AS.
- The user presents the TGT to the Ticket Granting Service (TGS) when requesting network service access.
- TGS creates a Service Ticket (ticket and session key) that user presents to network service for validation.

Authentication can also be based on digital certificates and are a preferred solution for integration with non-Windows systems.

The strongest authentication can be easily defeated through weak passwords. You can establish password policies that enforce password length, complexity, lifetime, and reversible encryption use and reuse. You can also define Account Lockout Policy as a means to help you detect and hopefully block attempts at unauthorized access to the network.

Scenario

In your discussions with representatives from the other Ready-Biz divisions, you discover that there is a need for direct access to data and other resources between divisions. This is being handled in an ad hoc manner, with a few users in each division authorized to create and delete trust relationships and assign access permissions on an as-needed basis. This has lead to a nearly incomprehensible mass of trusts crossing back and forth between domains, as well as assignment of unnecessary access permissions.

Another surprise from the other divisions is the existence of non-Windows systems. These include Unix-based DNS servers and Linux-based graphics workstations.

There is also a request for forest-wide administrators to be able to verify and correct, if necessary, security configurations in other divisions. There is a concern that other divisions might have a tendency to continue the status quo if not watched closely.

Representatives from each division have been brought together to define specific resource access and management requirements between divisions.

Lesson 7 Designing a Logical Authentication Strategy

Project	Exam 70-298 Objective
7.1 Designing Forest and Domain Trust Models	**Design a logical authentication strategy**. Design forest and domain trust models.
7.2 Designing Security to Meet Interoperability Requirements	**Design a logical authentication strategy**. Design security that meets interoperability requirements.
7.3 Establishing Account and Password Requirements	**Design a logical authentication strategy**. Establish account and password requirements for security.

General Requirements

To complete Project 7.3, you will need administrative rights on a Windows 2000, Windows XP Professional, or Windows Server 2003 computer. You may also find it helpful to refer to Lesson 7 in your Prentice Hall Certification Series Exam 70-298 textbook for additional information about the topics covered by the projects in this lesson.

project 7.1

Designing Forest and Domain Trust Models

exam objective

Design a logical authentication strategy. Design forest and domain trust models.

overview

From your discussions with other divisions, you now know that you need to modify the trust relationships in your security design. The design calls for controlling cross-forest access to resources through trust relationships and access permissions. You must determine if, and where, you need explicitly defined trust relationships. You must identify where you need to apply trusts between forests (**Figure 7-1**) and where you need to apply shortcut trusts directly between domains (**Figure 7-2**).

You basic access requirements are:

- United States forest-wide administrators need administrator access to all domains.
- Forest-wide administrators on other forest do not need administrator access to other forests.
- Users need access to files and printers hosted in other divisions.
- Warehouse departments must be able to directly compare and transfer inventory data.

Each division has a central warehouse configured as a separate domain. Warehouses connect to their parent networks through slower wide-area links than other offices.

learning objective

After completing this project, you will be more familiar with external trust relationships and trust relationship design.

specific requirements

None

estimated completion time

20 minutes

project steps

1. To ensure full functionality of trust relationship features, what configuration changes might be required in the existing forests?
2. What trust relationships are required to meet administrative requirements?
3. What trust relationships are required to meet user requirements?
4. How would you configure trust relationships between warehouses to optimize performance?
5. Using **Figure 5-3** as your base, sketch your trust relationship design. Include the direction of any one-way trust relationships.

Figure 7-1 Forest trust relationship

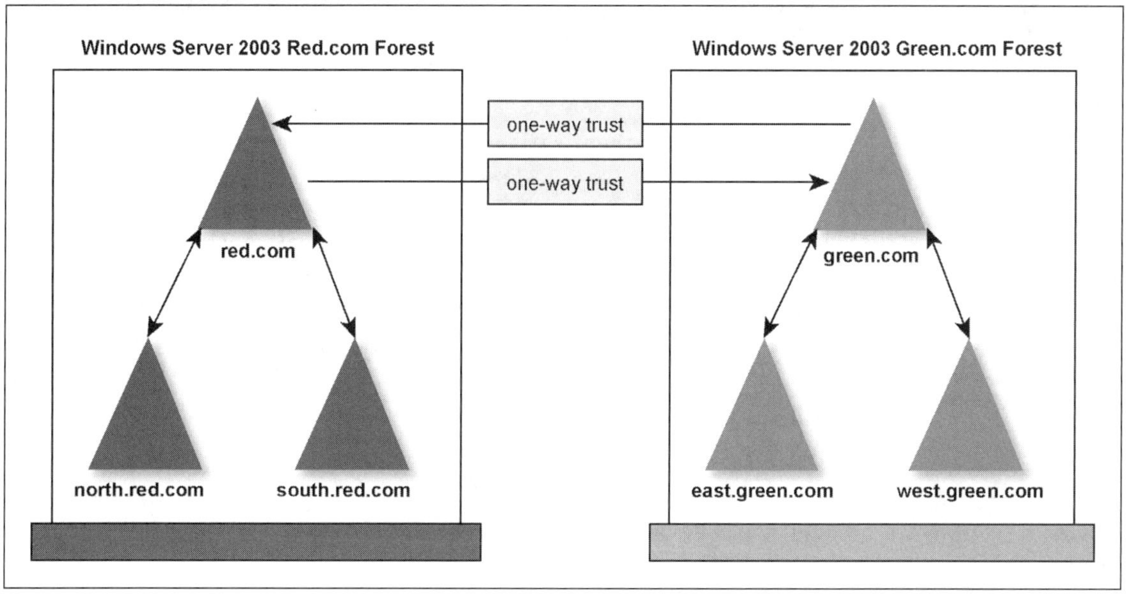

Figure 7-2 External trust relationship between Windows Server 2003 domains

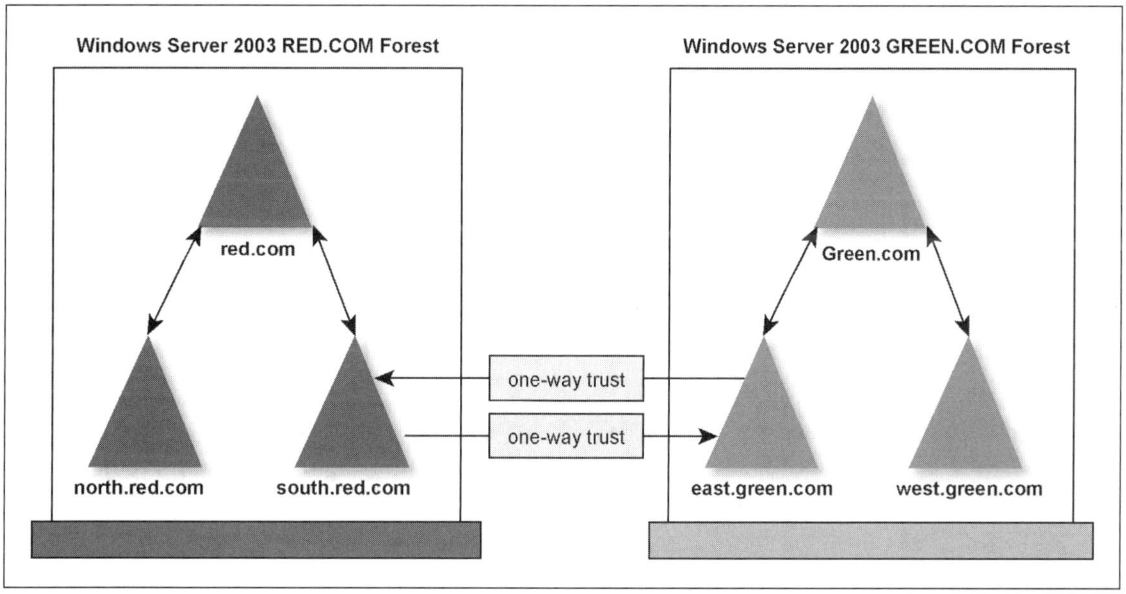

Figure 7-3 Ready-Biz domain model

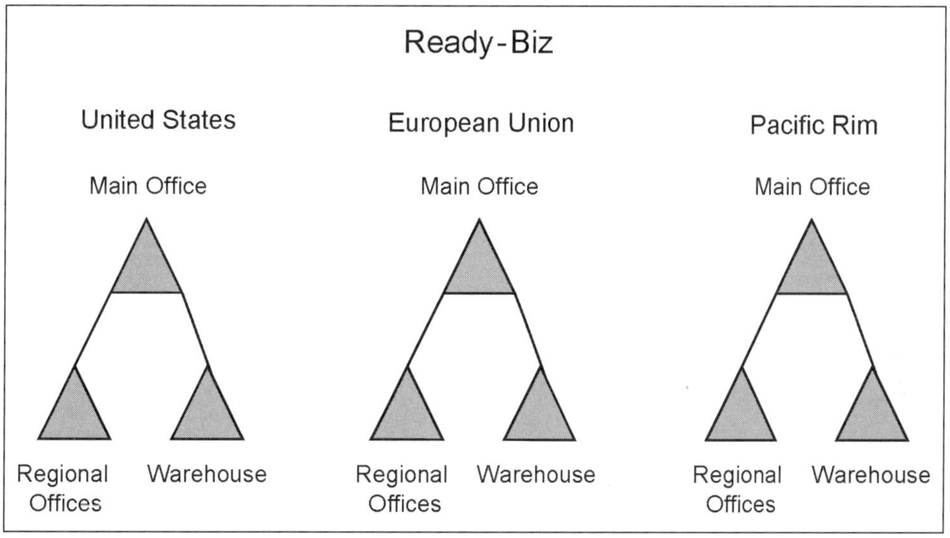

project 7.2

Designing Security to Meet Interoperability Requirements

exam objective

Design a logical authentication strategy. Design security that meets interoperability requirements.

overview

You are working directly with security personnel in all divisions to identify how authentication will be configured and how interoperability requirements will be met (**Table 7-1**). This is being done to ensure consistency when users access resources in other domains.

Review the mix of operating systems running on the network. Foreign divisions must also consider a small number of Unix machines. You have not yet seen a formal plan for replacing the Windows 95 computers.

learning objective

After completing this project, you will know how to identify authentication requirements by operating system.

specific requirements

None

estimated completion time

15 minutes

project steps

1. Identify all computers that will be able to use Kerberos v5. Include server and client systems.
2. Identify all computers that must use NTLMv2 authentication. Include server and client systems and any special configuration requirements.
3. As part of the background justification paperwork, prepare a short report comparing Kerberos v5 and NTLMv2. Refer to **Figure 7-4** and **Figure 7-5** to compare authentication methods.

Table 7-1 Authentication Protocols Supported By Operating System

Operating System	Authentication Protocols/Mechanisms Supported
Early Releases of Windows Operating Systems	
Windows 95/98	LAN Manager, remote access protocols, Web-based protocols
Windows 95/98 with Active Directory Services Client software installed	LAN Manager, NTLM, NTLMv2, remote access protocols, Web-based protocols
Windows NT 4 with Service Pack 4 or later	LAN Manager, NTLM, NTLMv2, certificates, remote access protocols, Web-based protocols
Current Releases of Windows Operating Systems	
Windows 2000	LAN Manager, NTLM, NTLMv2, certificates, Kerberos, remote access protocols, Web-based protocols
Windows Server 2003	LAN Manager, NTLM, NTLMv2, certificates, Kerberos, remote access protocols, Web-based protocols
Non-Windows Systems	
Unix	Kerberos, certificates, remote access protocols, Web-based protocols
Linux	Kerberos, certificates, remote access protocols, Web-based protocols
AS400	Kerberos, certificates, remote access protocols, Web-based protocols
Mainframes	Kerberos, certificates, remote access protocols, Web-based protocols

Figure 7-4 Challenge/response mechanism of NTLM

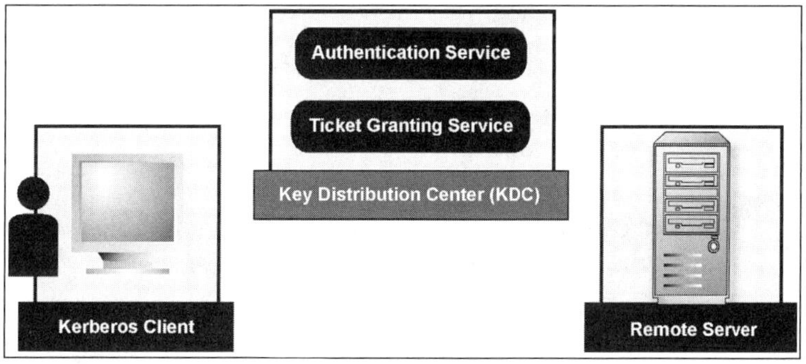

Figure 7-5 Kerberos v5 protocol authentication process

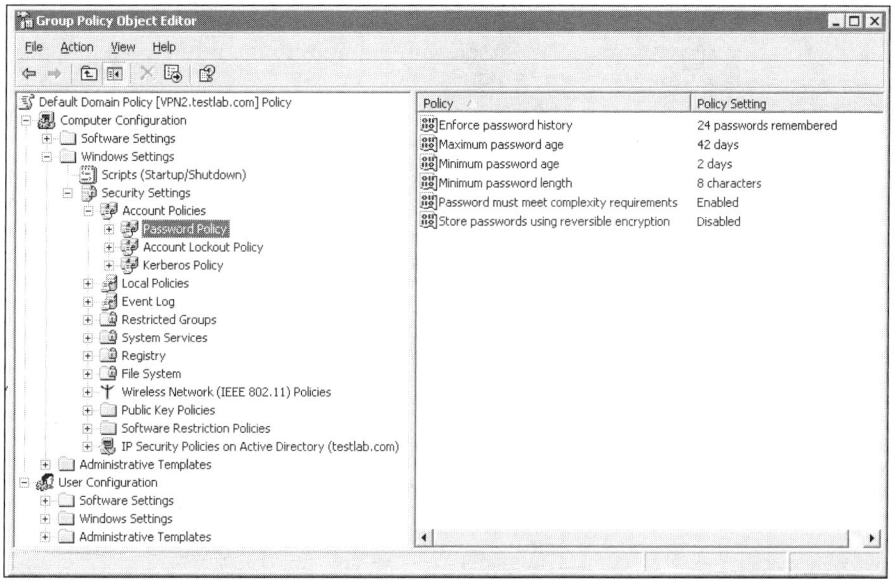

project 7.3

Establishing Account and Password Requirements

exam objective

Design a logical authentication strategy. Establish account and password requirements for security.

overview

The preferred security design calls for consistent password policies (**Table 7-2**) and account lockout policies throughout the company. Proposed standards include the following:

- Require complex passwords of seven (or more) characters.
- Change passwords every 30 days.
- Require one week between password changes.
- Remember the last 12 passwords.
- Do not allow reversible encryption.
- Lock user out after 3 failed attempts in 15 minutes.
- An administrator must unlock the account to make it available.

You do not know if all domains currently have consistent policies.

learning objective

After completing this project, you will know how to configure password and authentication to meet security design requirements.

specific requirements

See General Requirements.

estimated completion time

15 minutes

project steps

Check a computer at random to see the current policy settings before preparing your recommendations.

1. Select **Start** and then click **Control Panel** to open the Control Panel window.
2. Double-click **Administrative Tools** to open the **Administrative Tools** window.
3. Double-click **Local Security Policy** to open the **Local Security Settings** window.
4. Expand **Account Policy** in the left pane of the window.
5. Double-click **Password Policy** to review the current password policies. Prepare a short report comparing the current policy settings to the policies specified by the security design.
6. Close the Local Security Settings window.
7. How can you manage security policies from Chicago and ensure that password and account lockout policies are applied consistently throughout the company enterprise?

tip

These steps were performed on a Windows XP Professional computer. If the computer you use has a different operating system, some of the steps may vary.

Table 7-2 Password Policy settings for Windows Server 2003 default installation

Setting	Default Value /Range shown in parenthesis	Recommended Values	Explanation of Setting
Enforce Password History	1 (0-24)	24	This setting defines how many passwords are retained in history. If the setting is not configured, a user could reuse a password even if it has expired. Microsoft recommends setting this to the maximum of 24 passwords remembered.
Maximum Password Age	42 days (0-999)	42 days	This setting determines how long a user can use a password before it expires and they will be forced to change it. If you do not enable this setting, the user will be able to use a password indefinitely. If you configure this setting for passwords to expire too quickly, then users may start writing their passwords down on paper!
Minimum Password Age	0 days (0-299)	2 days	This setting can be used to prevent users from bypassing the enforcement of the password history and password expiration (password age) settings. For example, if this policy is not set, and Mary's password expires, she could change the password to a particular value a sufficient number of times that would allow her to return to her original password. Microsoft recommends setting this policy to two days.
Minimum Password Length	0 characters (0-14)	8 characters	This setting determines the minimum number of characters a user must include in their password. Be sure to educate users on how to create strong passwords. Microsoft recommends a minimum of eight characters.
Password Must Meet Complexity Requirements	Disabled (enabled/disabled)	Enabled	When this policy is enabled, passwords must include at least three of the following: uppercase letters, lowercase letters, numbers, and special symbols. Microsoft recommends enabling this policy.
Store Passwords Using Reversible Encryption	Disabled (enabled/disabled)	Disabled	This policy should be enabled when a domain controller needs to decrypt the password quickly when certain authentication protocols are used. For example, Challenge Handshake Authentication Protocol (CHAP). It is also used when Macintosh systems are included in the network. Because this setting can be set on individual user accounts, Microsoft recommends that you disable this policy for the domain unless it is required for everyone.

LESSON

8 Designing Network Infrastructure Security

Defending your network's perimeters from attack and securing data as it travels across your network are essential to ensuring that your network servers and the data they store are protected from intruders. You must design a strategy that allows legitimate traffic to be passed optimally across the network while reducing the potential attack surface at the perimeters and on key systems on the network. When designing a network security strategy, consider the following:

- Where are your network boundaries? Make sure to include remote access, virtual private network (VPN), and internal network segment boundaries.
- Which protocols must be supported on a network segment?
- Which protocols must be allowed to cross segments?
- What type of network security device is appropriate to guard each perimeter?
- Are there encryption requirements?
- Where are key infrastructure servers located?
- How is infrastructure traffic secured?

After you have answered these questions, you can begin to identify the devices and technologies you will use to protect legitimate traffic and to reduce the attack surface on your network. This means protecting both internal and external transmissions. Some technologies you might consider include the following:

- Firewalls
- Proxy servers
- Intrusion detection systems (IDSs)
- Intrusion protection systems (IPSs)
- Remote Authentication Dial-In User Service (RADIUS)
- Internet Protocol Security (IPSec)
- VPNs

Regardless of the technologies you choose, you must carefully design the policies that define their implementation. When configuring firewalls, you must determine which ports you will have to open to support network services and inter-site communications. Because each port represents a potential security hole, your design should open only those ports required, blocking traffic in the remaining Transmission Control Protocol (TCP) and User Datagram Protocol (UDP) ports.

One area that is sometimes overlooked in security design is the need to protect Domain Name System (DNS) servers. DNS servers are potentially susceptible to cache poisoning and Denial of Service (DoS) and Distributed DoS (DDoS) attacks. External name servers—those services name resolution requests by external users—are especially susceptible and must be considered in your design.

Scenario

You are working with a team made of up individuals from each of the offices in the United States to design the network security. The goal is to first design network security for the Chicago office, then implement a similar infrastructure at all other United States offices. You must also identify how traffic between the Chicago office and the offices in Europe and Asia will be secured. The following security requirements must be met by your design:

- Financial data must be encrypted on the network.
- Inter-site communication must be encrypted.
- No unsolicited traffic must enter the internal network from the Internet.
- Only the company's File Transfer Protocol (FTP) server should respond to FTP traffic.
- DNS traffic must be secured.

Lesson 8 Designing Network Infrastructure Security

Project	*Exam 70-298 Objective*
8.1 Introducing Network Perimeters and Devices	**Design network infrastructure security.**
8.2 Identifying the Required Protocols for a Firewall Configuration	**Design network infrastructure security**. Design network infrastructure security. Specify the required protocols for a firewall configuration.
8.3 Securing Internal Data Transmissions	**Design network infrastructure security**. Design security for data transmission. Design IP filtering. Design an IPSec Policy.
8.4 Securing Domain Name System (DNS) Service	**Design network infrastructure security**. Design network infrastructure security. Secure a DNS implementation.

General Requirements

There are no special requirements for this lesson. However, you may find it helpful to refer to Lesson 8 in your Prentice Hall Certification Series Exam 70-298 textbook for additional information about the topics covered by the projects in this lesson.

project 8.1

Introducing Network Perimeters and Devices

exam objective

Design network infrastructure security.

overview

You have identified three network perimeters at the Chicago office. The perimeters are shown in **Figure 8-1**. The company's Chicago domain controllers are located on the internal network segment, as is the e-mail server. The Web server, FTP server, and virtual private network end-point are located on the screened subnet.

You must make recommendations for protecting each segment.

learning objective

After completing this project, you will be able to identify the most appropriate network security device to address a given requirement.

specific requirements

None

estimated completion time

15 minutes

project steps

1. Prepare a PowerPoint or other form of presentation that identifies the most appropriate type of firewall to position at the following perimeters:
   - Internet/screened subnet
   - Screened subnet/internal network

   Support your recommendations by citing required features.
2. What benefit would be gained by including an intrusion protection system (IPS) on the subnet that contains the financial servers?
3. The FTP server stores some company-confidential data. What step can you take to further secure the FTP server, while still allowing access from the Internet?

Figure 8-1 Ready-Biz network perimeters

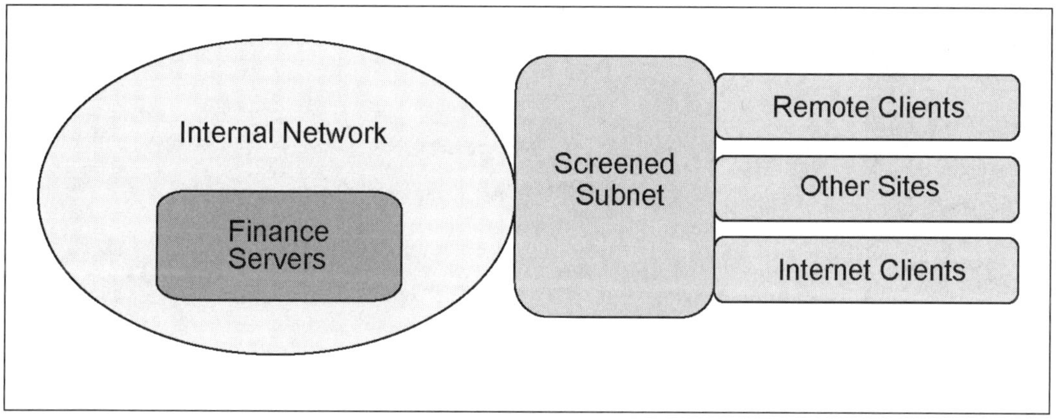

project 8.2

Identifying the Required Protocols for a Firewall Configuration

exam objective

Design network infrastructure security. Design network infrastructure security. Specify the required protocols for a firewall configuration.

overview

Now that you have identified the devices that will guard the border between the Internet and the screened subnet as well as the border between the screened subnet and the perimeter network, you must identify the protocols that will be used by each device that the ports that must be opened up to, to allow necessary inter-site and intra-site communication.

You have been asked to identify the protocols that are required to support Active Directory replication between sites. As you'll recall, the United States offices are implemented as a single forest, with the root domain in Chicago. Each site is implemented as its own domain **(Figure 8-2)**. A domain controller for each domain is located in the Chicago office.

You must determine the best replication protocol to use and the most secure way to implement it.

learning objective

After completing this project, you will understand how to configure secure replication across firewalls.

specific requirements

None

estimated completion time

10 minutes

project steps

1. Which replication protocol will you use for replication between the Chicago site and a regional office site?
2. What is the most secure way to implement replication between the Chicago site and a regional office site?
3. Create a document that identifies the ports that must be opened in the firewalls to support replication between the Chicago site and a regional office site.
4. Which replication protocol will you use for replication between two regional office sites?

Figure 8-2 Active Directory design

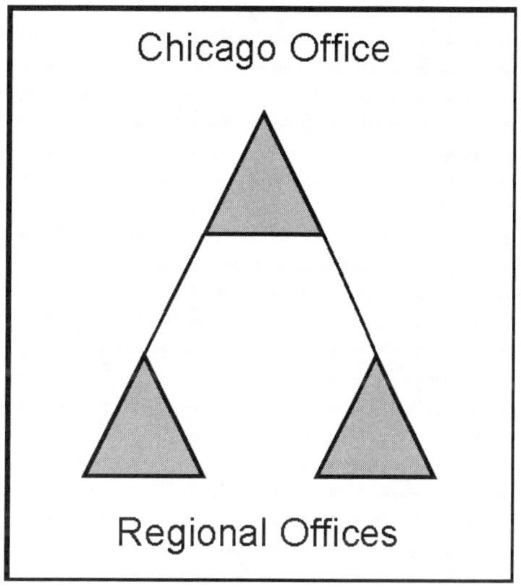

project 8.3

Securing Internal Data Transmissions

exam objective

Design network infrastructure security. Design security for data transmission. Design IP filtering. Design an IPSec Policy.

overview

Several security requirements can be met by using IPSec. These requirements include the following:

- Financial data must be encrypted on the network. Only domain members will access financial data.
- Inter-site communication must be encrypted.
- Only the company's FTP server should respond to FTP traffic.

You must design IPSec policies to meet each of these requirements. **Figure 8-3** shows the components of an IPSec policy.

It is your job to analyze each of the above requirements and design the necessary rules to meet each requirement.

learning objective

After completing this project, you will know how to design an IPSec policy to meet requirements.

specific requirements

None

estimated completion time

15 minutes

project steps

1. Design an IPSec policy that requires data sent to and from the financial servers to be encrypted on the network. Identify the following:
   - Will the policy use transport or tunnel mode?
   - Which filter action will you use?
   - Which authentication method will you use?
   - Will you use Authentication Header, Encapsulating Security Protocol, or both?
2. Design an IPSec policy that requires inter-site communication to be encrypted:
   - Will the policy use transport or tunnel mode?
   - Which filter action will you use?
   - Which authentication method will you use between sites in the United States?
   - Which authentication method will you use between a site in the United States and a site in Europe?
3. Design an IPSec policy that prevents all computers except the FTP server from responding to FTP requests:
   - Which filter action will you use?
   - Is an authentication method required?

Figure 8-3 IP Security policy components

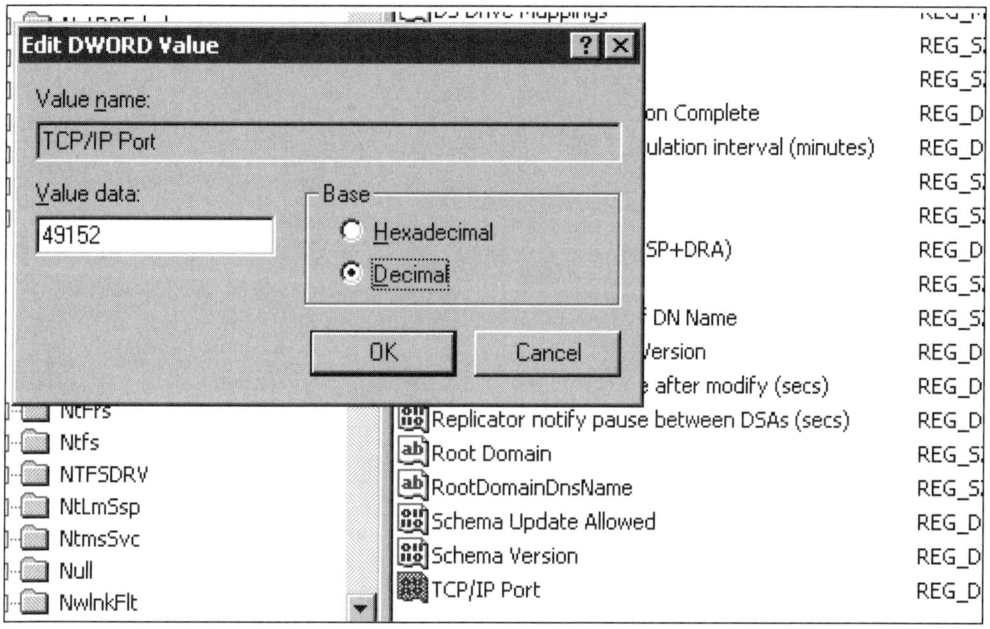

project 8.4

Securing Domain Name System (DNS) Service

exam objective

Design network infrastructure security. Design network infrastructure security. Secure a DNS implementation.

overview

When Ready-Biz upgraded the Chicago domain from Windows NT 4 to Windows Server 2003, the DNS server on the screened subnet was upgraded to Windows Server 2003 and configured to allow dynamic updates. The regional offices have DNS servers in their screened subnets. Some of these DNS servers run Windows Server 2003. Others run Windows NT 4 or, in some limited cases, Unix.

The DNS server at each location is configured with a primary zone for the domain implemented at that location and a secondary zone for each other domain in the United States. **Figure 8-4** shows potential vulnerabilities with the current DNS system.

You must design a secure DNS implementation that allows for dynamic updates for internal clients, but still allows clients to access Internet resources.

learning objective

After completing this project, you will know how to secure a DNS implementation.

specific requirements

None

estimated completion time

10 minutes

project steps

1. How will you restructure the DNS implementation at the Chicago office?
2. What type of zone will you create to resolve the names for internal resources?
3. What step will you take to allow users on the internal to network resolve the names for servers on the screened subnet?
4. What steps must you take before you can eliminate zone transfer traffic between the internal DNS server in Chicago and the internal DNS server at each regional office?

Figure 8-4 Common attacks against DNS servers

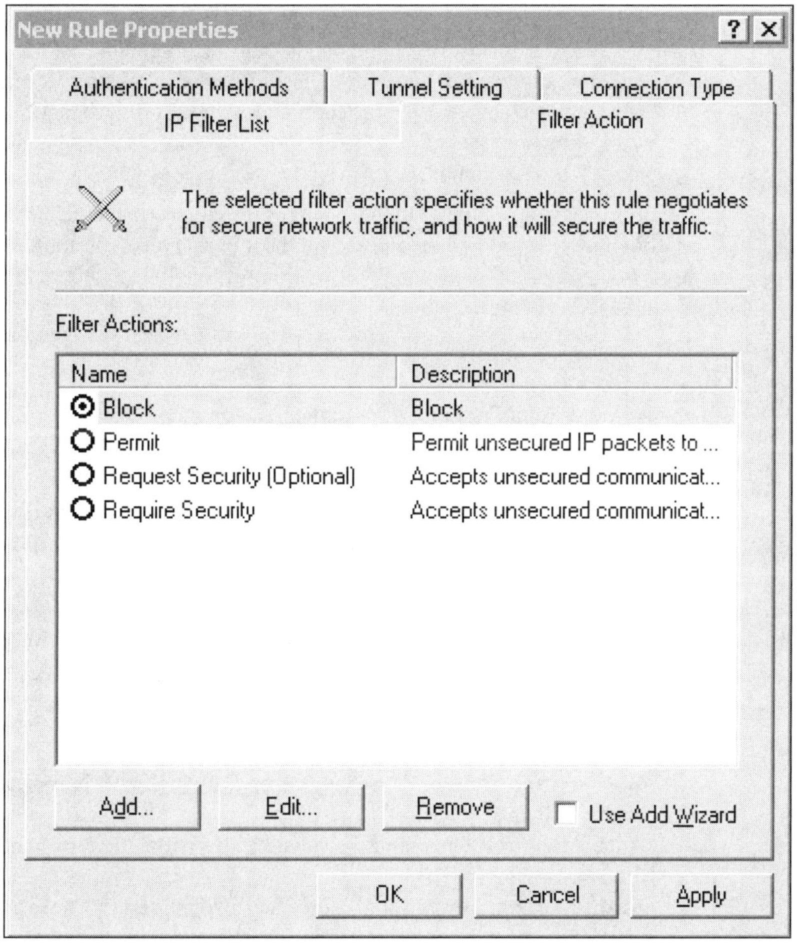

LESSON

9 Designing Security for Communication Between Networks

Lesson 8 introduced components and technologies for secure intra- and inter-network communications. Designing secure communications requires determining how best to configure and deploy these communications. Communication security design focuses around the use of virtual private networks (VPNs), but the wide variety of configuration and implementation options means that communication design is no simple task.

You must decide the type of tunnel used for the connection, either voluntary (created by the client) or compulsory (created and required by the VPN server). You must choose the tunneling protocol used to communicate, either Point-to-Point Tunneling Protocol (PPTP) or Layer 2 Tunneling Protocol (L2TP).

PPTP features include:

- IP network required.
- Point-to-Point Protocol (PPP) authentication methods.
- Link encryption (only) using Microsoft Point-to-Point Encryption (MPPE) protocol.
- No support for data integrity, data origin authentication, or delivery confirmation.

L2TP is a more secure communication option, with features including:

- IP networks, Asynchronous Transfer Mode (ATM), Frame Relay, and X.25 support.
- Authentication by certificate or pre-shared keys.
- End-to-end encryption using IPSec.
- Support for data integrity, data origin authentication, and delivery configuration.

Either PPTP or L2TP, the tunnel and a control connection must be established before encrypted data transmission.

When configuring VPN connectivity, concerns include:

- **VPN servers:** Determining the number and type of VPN servers, as well as where they are deployed in the network.
- **Authentication:** Choosing the most secure authentication method(s) while supporting all necessary client types.
- **Authorization:** Set through rules defined in remote access policy and through client properties.
- **Encryption:** Encryption type depends on tunnel protocol, but you can still configure encryption levels and requirements.

Firewall configuration, input and output filters, will depend on your VPN protocol and the VPN server physical location.

If a full-time connection is not required, VPN connections can be configured to use demand-dial routing. Along with the connection information, it is necessary to configure the authentication type and authorization through connection properties and remote access policy.

There might also be a need to configure access to your network for outside organizations. This requires digital certificates from a CA trusted by the computers at each end of the tunnel. The best solution is to have the client and VPN server use certificates from the same CA, or from issuing CAs with the same root CA. Often, the companies at each end will purchase certificates from a public CA. However, a private CA can be used, as long as it is trusted by and accessible to each of the parties.

Scenario

You are continuing to design network communication requirements. You've prepared a basic design specification that includes:

- All offices in a division connect to the main office.
- Each main office connects directly all other main divisional offices.

The connection to the main office will be a full-time connection, as are the connections between the main offices. You have been asked to evaluate some additional connection options. The overriding concern on all connections is data security.

Lesson 9 Designing Security for Communication Between Networks	
Project	***Exam 70-298 Objective***
9.1 Introducing Protocols Used for VPN Access	**Design security for communication between networks**. Select protocols for VPN access.
9.2 Examining VPN Connectivity	**Design security for communication between networks**. Design VPN connectivity.
9.3 Understanding Demand-Dial Routing Between Networks	**Design security for communication between networks**. Design demand-dial routing between internal networks.
9.4. Securing Communications with External Organizations	**Design security for communication between networks**. Design security for communication with external organizations. Design an extranet infrastructure.

General Requirements

There are no special requirements for this lesson. However, you may find it helpful to refer to Lesson 9 in your Prentice Hall Certification Series Exam 70-298 textbook for further information about the topics covered by the projects in this lesson.

project 9.1

Introducing Protocols Used for VPN Access

exam objective

Design security for communication between networks. Select protocols for VPN access.

overview

You must identify the requirements for the preferred communication configurations. This includes the use of compulsory tunnels for connections between offices **(Figure 9-1)** and voluntary tunnels for remote client connections **(Figure 9-2)**.

learning objective

After completing this project, you will understand differences between the PPTP and L2TP tunneling protocols.

specific requirements

None

estimated completion time

10 minutes

project steps

1. Compare PPTP and L2TP security features. Prepare a recommendation for the most secure connection option. Justify the recommendation with specific feature examples.
2. As part of your background reference materials for the security design, describe the requirements for secure, automated authentication between offices **(Figure 9-3)**.

Figure 9-1 Site-to-site (compulsory) VPN tunnel

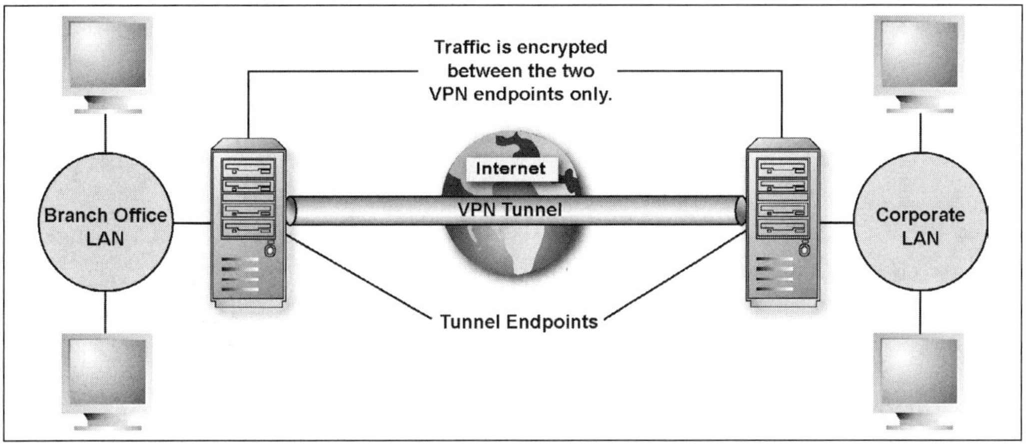

Figure 9-2 Remote access (voluntary) VPN tunnel

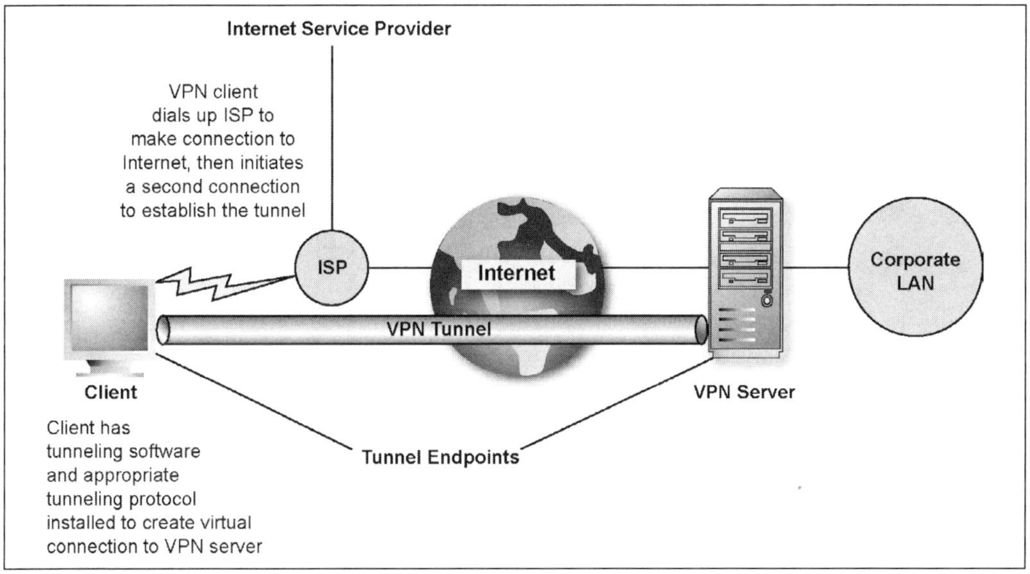

Figure 9-3 L2TP over IPSec using certificates to establish security association

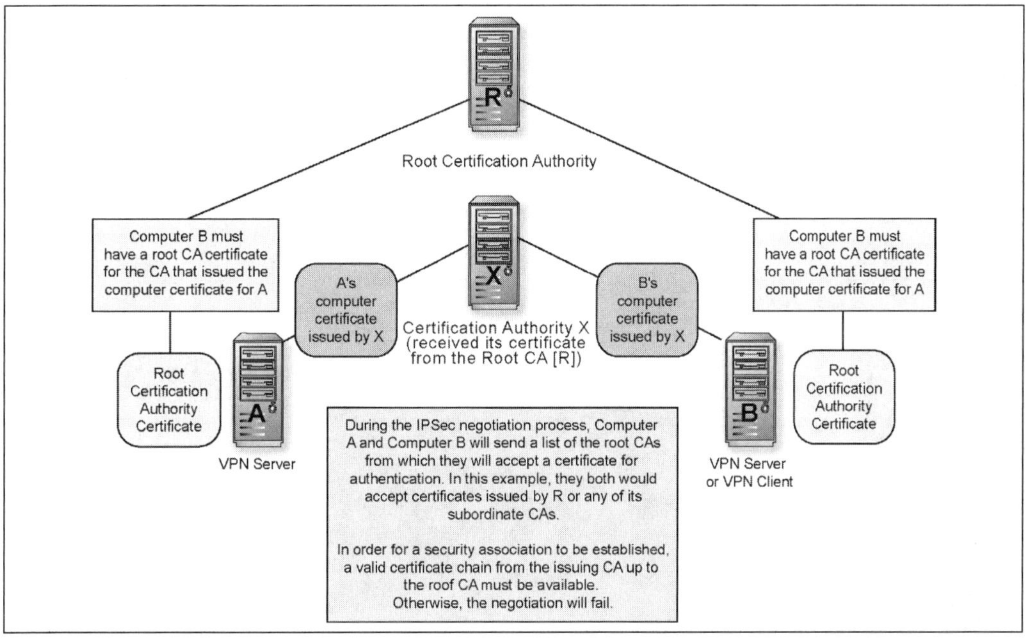

project 9.2

Examining VPN Connectivity

exam objective

Design security for communications between networks. Design VPN connectivity.

overview

You are continuing the design for connectivity between offices. You must determine the most appropriate placement for VPN servers **(Figure 9-4)**. You must:

- Provide optimum protection against unauthorized access from the Internet.
- Isolate the VPN server(s) from the internal network.

You must also design connectivity between main offices to minimize the chance of link failures. The primary concern is that the connection remains available unless a catastrophic failure occurs.

learning objective

After completing this project, you will understand VPN server placement options and multiple VPN server configurations.

specific requirements

None

estimated completion time

15 minutes

project steps

1. What is the most appropriate placement for the VPN servers used to connect offices? Justify your selection.
2. Compare DNS round-robin **(Figure 9-5)** and clustering **(Figure 9-6)**:
   - What features are similar?
   - What features are different?
   - Which configuration is best suited to your requirement?

Figure 9-4 VPN server placement

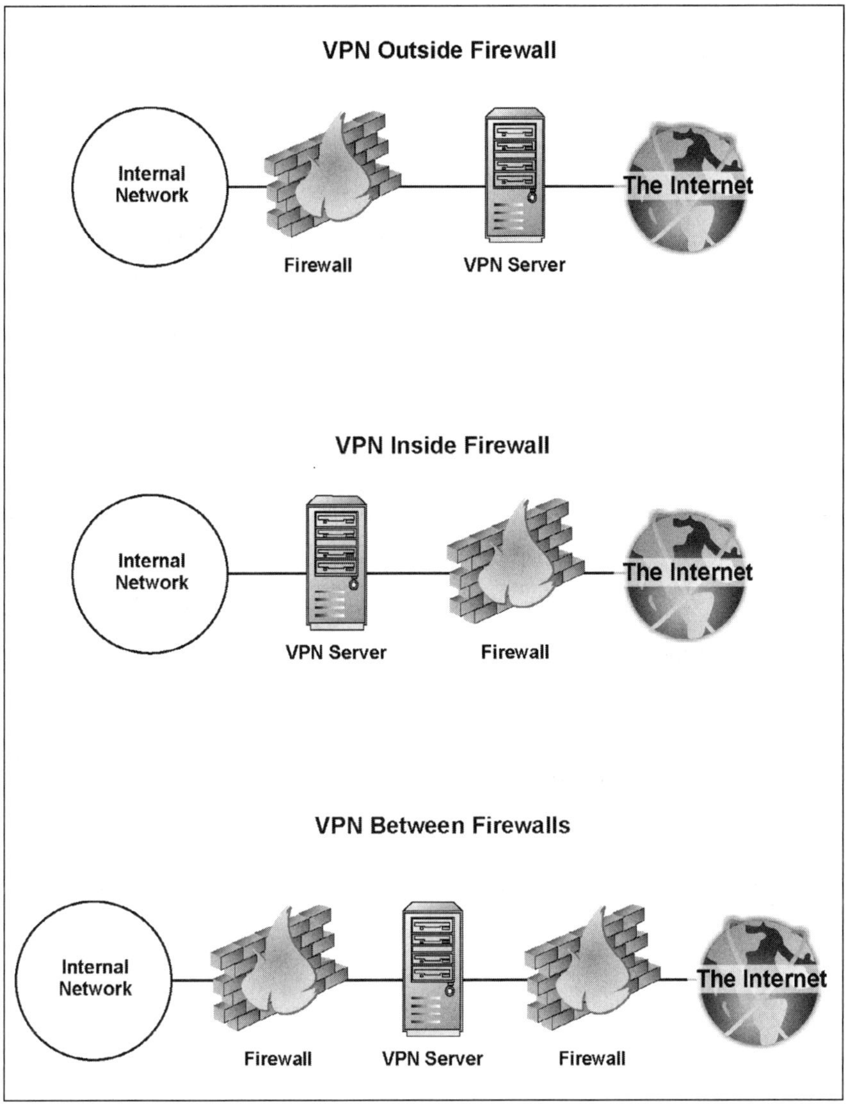

Figure 9-5 DNS round-robin solution for load balancing VPN servers

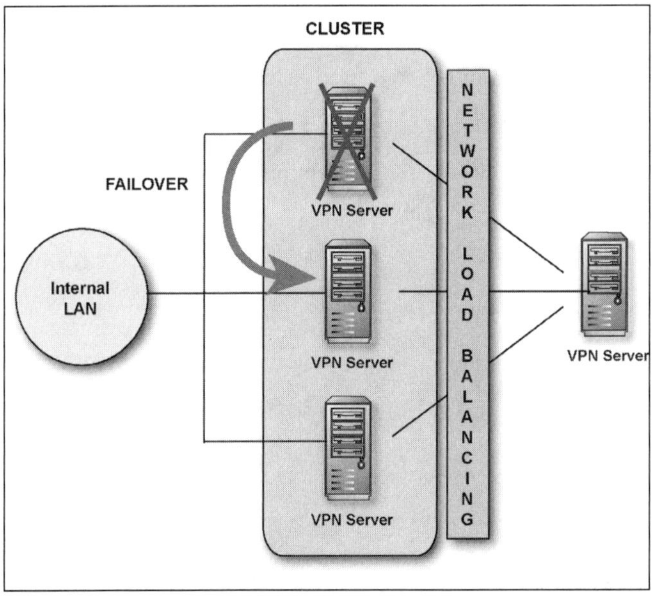

Figure 9-6 Clustering solutions for VPN servers

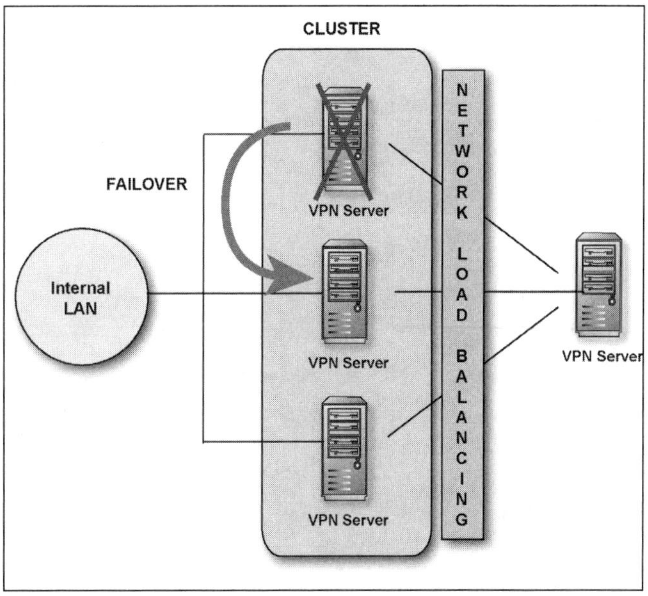

project 9.3

Understanding Demand-Dial Routing Between Networks

exam objective

Design security for communications between networks. Design demand-dial routing between internal networks.

overview

You are informed that the inventory control system is being updated to provide current inventory information and better control of the just-in-time manufacturing processes. Currently, a SQL Server 2000 server database at each warehouse tracks inventory for that warehouse only. The information for all warehouses will be combined into a single, horizontally partitioned database. The database will have the entire company inventory, identified by the warehouse in which it is stored.

Each warehouse office will have a copy of the combined databases. Users at the warehouse will be able to directly modify inventory information of the local warehouse only. Other changes are made through distributed transactions processed by the individual warehouse servers.

The warehouses will update each other through merge replication. The merge replication traffic will be encrypted between offices, but does not need to be locally encrypted. Because of the limited bandwidth between the warehouses and other offices, the replication traffic should not be allowed to impact other network traffic, so the offices will have to connect directly to each other. Each office will update the other two warehouses in a mesh configuration (**Figure 9-7**). Periodic connections should be used, connecting only on an as-needed basis (**Figure 9-8**).

learning objective

After completing this project, you will understand requirements for configuring demand-dial routing configurations.

specific requirements

None, but you will need to reference technologies discussed in Project 9.1 and Project 9.2.

estimated completion time

15 minutes

project steps

1. What is the minimum number of VPN servers required in each warehouse office to support replication?
2. Under the current specifications, which tunneling protocol(s) can you use?
3. If the specification changes to require point-to-point encryption between the SQL Server 2000 servers, which tunneling protocol(s) can you use?

Figure 9-7 Warehouse communication configuration

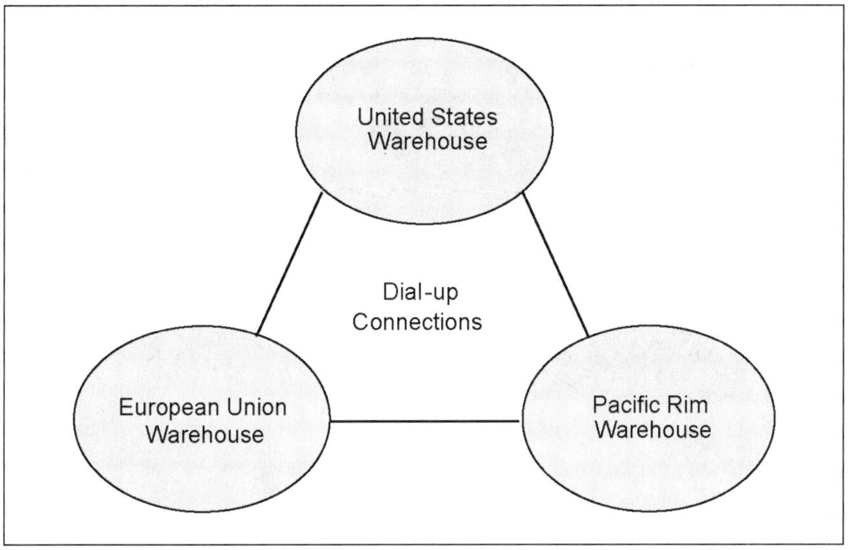

Figure 9-8 Dial-up VPN connection

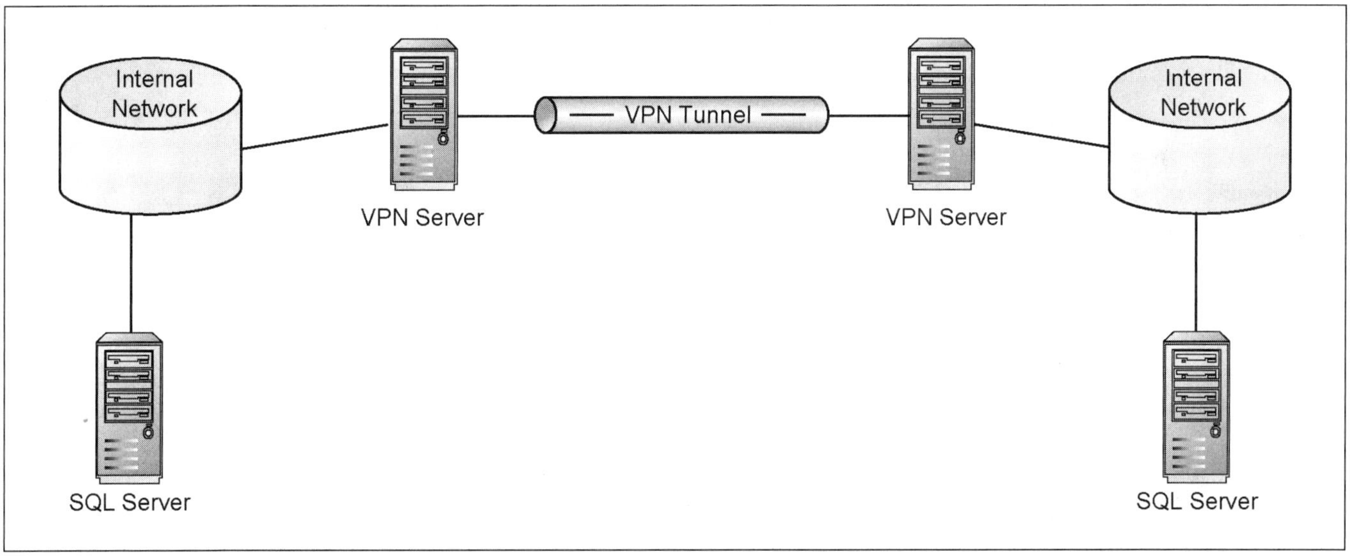

project 9.4

Securing Communications with External Organizations

exam objective

Design security for communications between networks. Design security for communication with external networks. Design an extranet infrastructure.

overview

One of the long-term business goals is increasing the use of business-to-business (B2B) technologies to improve efficiency and to cut costs. Although not part of the first phase of the security upgrades, you are asked to identify connectivity requirements to implement this.

learning objective

After completing this project, you will understand requirements for connecting with external organizations.

specific requirements

None

estimated completion time

10 minutes

project steps

1. As part of the background documentation for the security design, describe the process of mutual authentication between external organizations **(Figure 9-9)**.
2. What would be needed to provide certificates for authentication?
3. Explain why you would not use a local enterprise CA in this situation.

Figure 9-9 Mutual authentication between external organizations

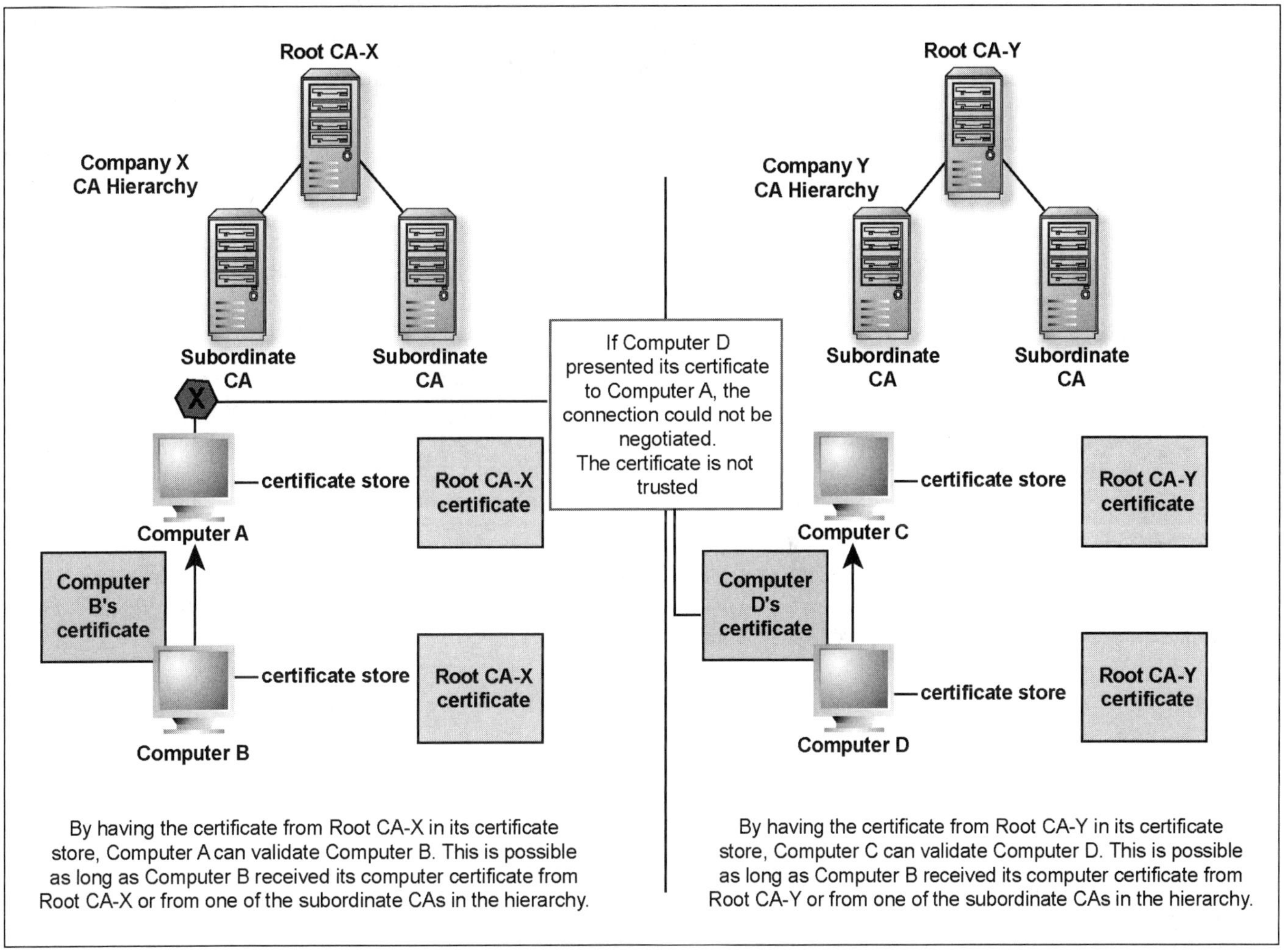

LESSON

10 Designing Security Based on Server Roles

In most network environments, there are a number of servers, each of which performs a specific role. In some cases, a server might perform multiple roles. One example of this is a domain controller that is also a DNS server (Other common roles include acting as a Dynamic Host Configuration Protocol [DHCP] server, a Windows Internet Name Service [WINS] server, and a Remote Access Service [RAS] server.) In other cases, a server performs only one role. Regardless of how roles are divided between servers, it is essential that all servers in the environment be protected with appropriate security measures.

Many, but not all, security policies can be implemented through security templates and Group Policy. Policies that apply to all servers in the environment should be implemented using a baseline template. Baseline templates should define very strict settings that can be loosened by incremental templates. For example, you might disable the Print Spooler service in the baseline template and enable it only in the incremental template that is applied to print servers.

Security templates can be applied to a computer's Local Security Policy by using either Security Configuration and Analysis or Secedit. Security templates can be applied to domain members by importing the policy into a Group Policy Object (GPO) and linking the GPO to the appropriate container.

Scenario

You are working with a team made of up individuals from each of the offices in the United States to design the network security. The goal is to first design network security for the Chicago office, then implement a similar infrastructure at all other United States offices.

You must define a strategy for implementing security policy settings based on server roles. The following policies must be implemented on all servers:

- All non-essential services must be disabled.
- Only members of the Administrators group can change the startup mode for a service.
- Users must log on to a domain using complex passwords.
- The Guest account must be disabled on all servers.
- Only members of Administrators can log on interactively to a domain controller.
- Only members of Administrators and Server Operators can log on interactively to other servers.
- The Administrators group must be limited to members of the Domain Admins group.
- Client security requirements, with the exception of account security, have not been defined.

Lesson 10 Designing Security Based on Server Roles

Project	Exam 70-298 Objective
10.1 Introducing Security Templates and Tools	**Design security for servers that have specific roles**. Roles include domain controllers, network infrastructure server, file server, IIS server, terminal server, and POP3 mail server.
10.2 Using Baseline Security Templates	**Design security for servers that have specific roles**. Roles include domain controllers, network infrastructure server, file server, IIS server, terminal server, and POP3 mail server. Define a baseline security template for all systems.
10.3 Using Incremental Security Templates	**Design security for servers that have specific roles**. Roles include domain controllers, network infrastructure server, file server, IIS server, terminal server, and POP3 mail server. Create a plan to modify baseline security templates according to role.

General Requirements

To complete the projects in this lesson, you will need administrative rights on a Windows XP Professional or Windows Server 2003 computer. You may also find it helpful to refer to Lesson 10 in your Prentice Hall Certification Series Exam 70-298 textbook for additional information about the topics covered by the projects in this lesson.

project 10.1

Introducing Security Templates and Tools

exam objective

Design security for servers that have specific roles. Roles include domain controllers, network infrastructure server, file server, IIS server, terminal server, and POP3 mail server.

overview

You are evaluating the predefined security templates to determine what modifications would be necessary to use them as a baseline template. You will use the Security Configuration and Analysis snap-in to evaluate several of the security templates against your computer's current configuration.

As you'll recall, a policy setting is shown with a different icon, depending on its state (**Figure 10-1**). The icons are as follows:

- **Green check in a white circle:** The setting on the computer and the setting in the database are the same.
- **Red x:** The policy is configured in the database and on the computer, but the settings do not match.
- **Question mark:** The entry is not defined in the database, or the user does not have sufficient rights to perform the analysis.
- **Exclamation point:** The entry is defined in the database, but not on the computer.
- **No highlight:** The entry is not defined in the database or on the computer.

learning objective

After completing this project, you will know how to analyze a computer's security settings against those defined in one or more templates.

specific requirements

See General Requirements.

estimated completion time

15 minutes

project steps

1. Click **Start** and then click **Run** to open the **Run** dialog box.
2. Type **mmc** in the **Open** text box and then click **OK** to open an empty **Microsoft Management Console (MMC)**.
3. Click **File** on the **Menu** bar and then click **Add/Remove Snap-in**.
4. In the **Add/Remove Snap-in** dialog box, click **Add**.
5. The **Add Standalone Snap-in** dialog box opens. Select **Security Configuration and Analysis**, click **Add** and then click **Close**.
6. Click **OK** to close the Add/Remove Snap-in dialog box.
7. Right-click **Security Configuration and Analysis** in the left pane of the **Console Root** window and then click **Open Database**.
8. The **Open database** dialog box appears. Name the database **TemplateTest** and click **Open**.
9. The **Import Template** dialog box opens. Select **securews.inf** and click **Open**.
10. The **Console Root** window reappears. Right-click **Security Configuration and Analysis** in the right pane of the window and then click **Analyze Computer Now**.
11. The **Perform Analysis** dialog box opens. Click **OK** to confirm the default path for the error log.
12. After the analysis is performed, the **Console Root** window reappears. Click **Account Policies** to expand it and then choose **Password Policy**.

Figure 10-1 Results of analysis using the Security Configuration and Analysis snap-in

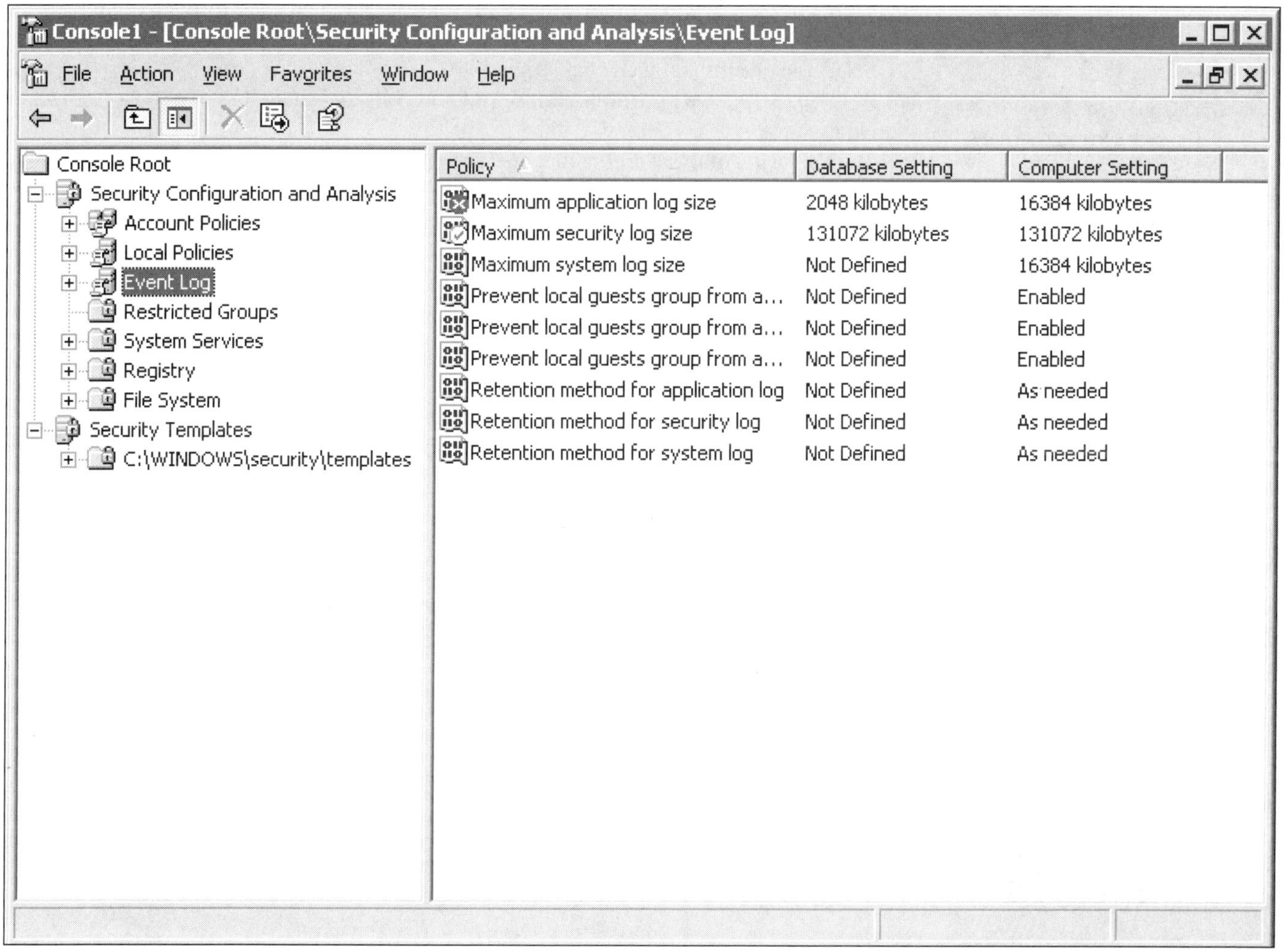

project 10.1

Introducing Security Templates and Tools *(cont'd)*

exam objective

Design security for servers that have specific roles. Roles include domain controllers, network infrastructure server, file server, IIS server, terminal server, and POP3 mail server.

project steps

13. Record the changes that will be made to the computer if the template is applied.
14. Go through each node and note the changes that would be made to the computer if the computer were configured with the template.
15. Select **File System** in the right pane of the **Console Root** window. Note that file system permissions were not analyzed.
16. Right-click **Security Configuration and Analysis** and then click **Import Template**. The **Import Template** dialog box opens **(Figure 10-2)**.
17. Select r**ootsec.inf** and then click **Open**.
18. Right-click **Security Configuration and Analysis** and then click **Analyze Computer Now**.
19. The **Perform Analysis dialog box** opens **(Figure 10-3)**. Click **OK** to confirm the default path for the error log.
20. Click **Password Policy** to view the settings and verify that the same changes are noted as you recorded in Step 14.
21. Select **File System**. Notice that the permissions on drive **C** were analyzed.
22. Close the console. Do not save changes.

Figure 10-2 **The Import Template dialog box**

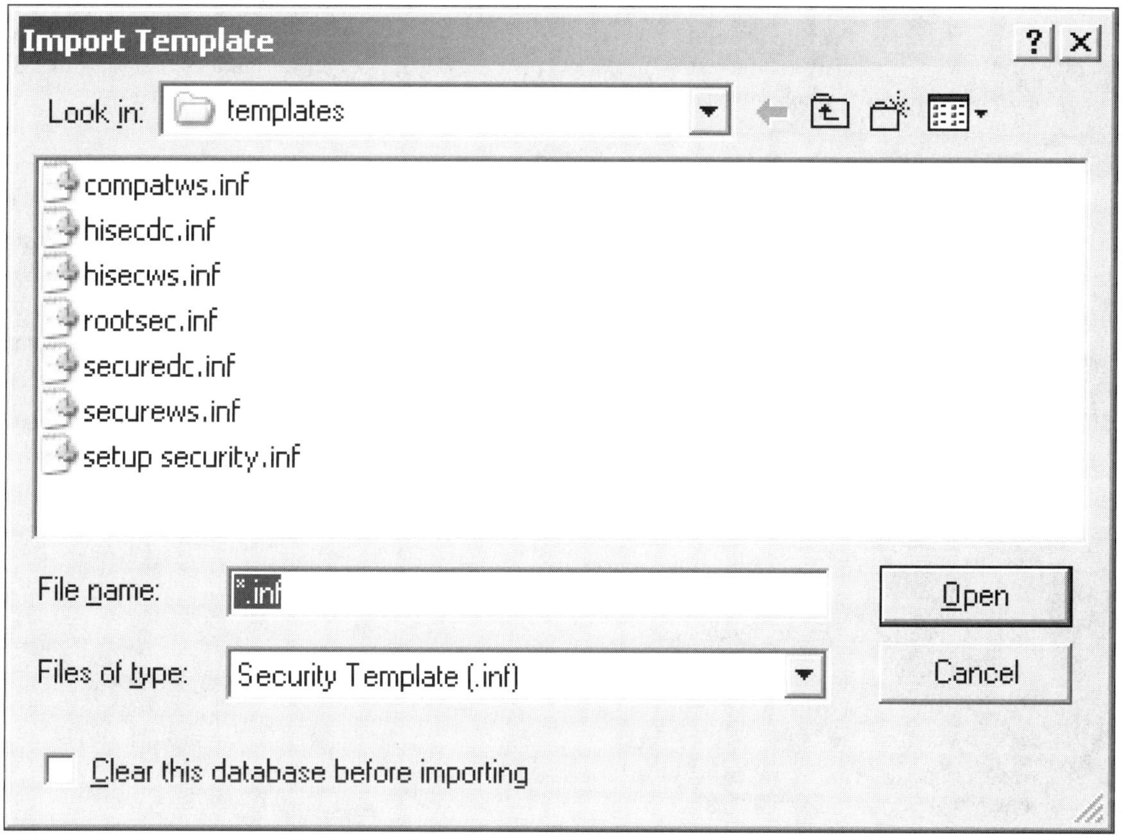

Figure 10-3 **The Perform Analysis dialog box**

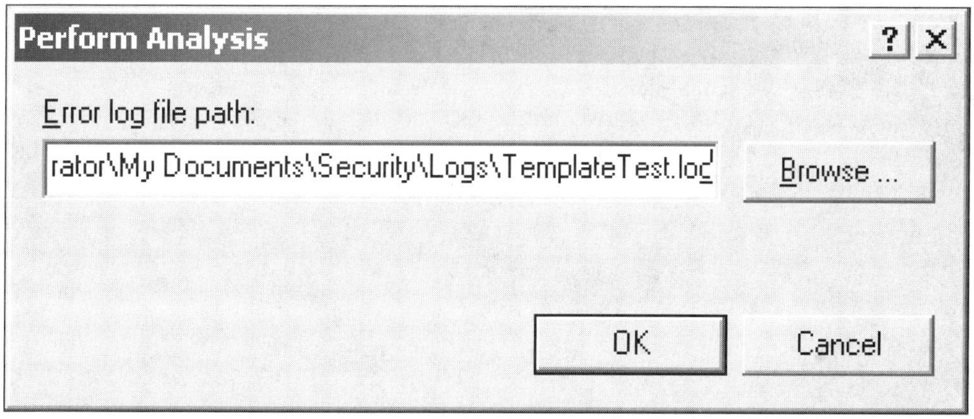

project 10.2 Using Baseline Security Templates

exam objective

Design security for servers that have specific roles. Roles include domain controllers, network infrastructure server, file server, IIS server, terminal server, and POP3 mail server. Define a baseline security template for all systems.

overview

You must analyze the security requirements of all servers and those of specific servers and design an organizational unit (OU) hierarchy that will allow you to configure those servers using baseline and incremental templates. As you'll recall, GPOs are processed according to the order of precedence shown in **Figure 10-4**.

When designing the strategy, you must consider the security requirements of various server roles. Some of these roles are shown in **Figure 10-5**. You must also consider the following requirements:

- File servers in Finance require stricter file permissions.
- All internal DNS servers are configured to use Active Directory to store zone information.
- Web servers and external DNS servers are not domain members.

learning objective

After completing this project, you will understand how to deploy baseline and incremental security templates.

specific requirements

None

estimated completion time

15 minutes

project steps

1. Design an OU hierarchy that will meet your requirements.
2. Where will you link a GPO with the security settings that should be applied to domain controllers?
3. Where will you link a GPO that enables the DNS service?
4. Where will you link the GPO that contains the baseline security template for all servers?
5. Where will you link the GPO that defines the password policy?

Figure 10-4 GPO order of precedence

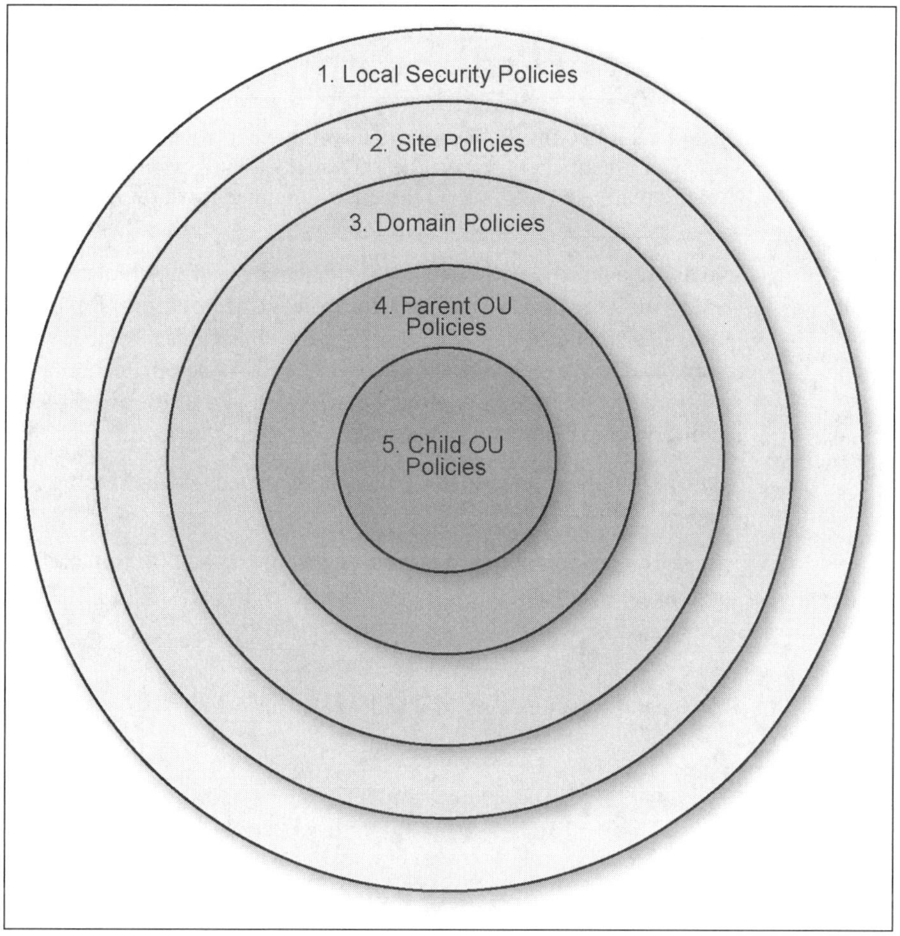

Figure 10-5 Server roles

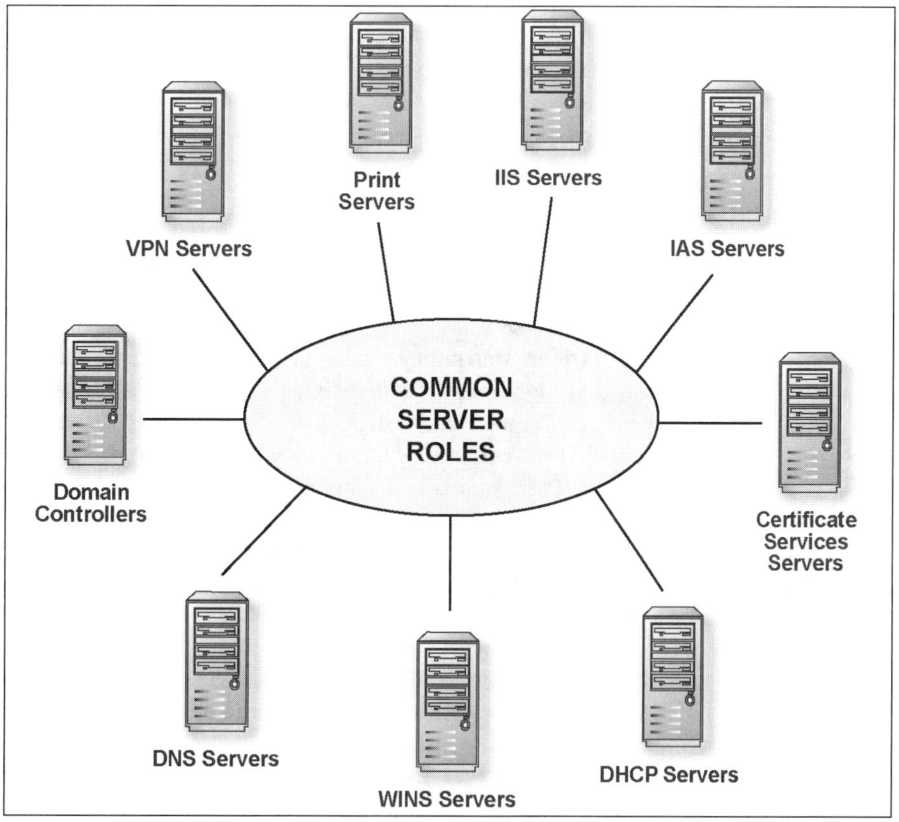

project 10.3

Using Incremental Security Templates

exam objective

Design security for servers that have specific roles. Roles include domain controllers, network infrastructure server, file server, IIS server, terminal server, and POP3 mail server. Create a plan to modify baseline security templates according to role.

overview

You are designing the baseline and incremental security templates to be used to configure the servers at Ready-Biz. You need to modify the securews.inf baseline template to meet requirements. One of the requirements is that unnecessary services must be disabled. You will disable the Print Spooler service. As you'll recall, incremental templates are used to override settings defined in the baseline template, as shown in **Figure 10-6**. You must also create an incremental template that enables the Print Spooler service.

You will import both templates into a database and test the result.

learning objective

After completing this project, you will know how to design and implement baseline and incremental templates.

specific requirements

See General Requirements. You should also have completed Project 10.1.

estimated completion time

15 minutes

project steps

1. Open an empty **MMC** console.
2. Add the **Security Templates** snap-in and the **Security Configuration and Analysis** snap-in.
3. Expand **Security Templates** in the left pane of the **Console Root** window.
4. Expand **C:\Windows\security\templates** in the left pane of the Console Root window.
5. Right-click **securews** and then click **Save As**.
6. The **Save As** dialog box opens. Name the template **baseline** and click **Save**.
7. The baseline template now appears under **C:\Windows\security\templates**. Click it to expand it.
8. Click **System Services**.
9. Double-click the **Print Spooler** service. The **Print Spooler Properties** dialog box appears.
10. Select the **Define this policy setting in the template** check box.
11. The **Security for Print Spooler** dialog box appears (**Figure 10-7**). Leave the security settings as they appear and click **OK**.
12. Verify that **Disabled** is selected in the **Select service startup mode** section of the Print Spooler Properties dialog box. Click **OK**.
13. Right-click **baseline** and then click **Save**.
14. Right-click **C:\Windows\security\templates** and choose **New Template**. The **C:\Windows\security\templates** dialog box opens.
15. Name the template **PrintServer** and click **OK**.
16. Modify the PrintServer template to configure the startup mode of the Print Spooler service to **Automatic**. To do so, expand the template, select **System Services**, open the **Print Spooler Properties** dialog box, and select the **Automatic** option button in the **Select service startup mode** section.
17. Right-click **PrintServer** and click **Save**.

Figure 10-6 Incremental template overrides baseline template

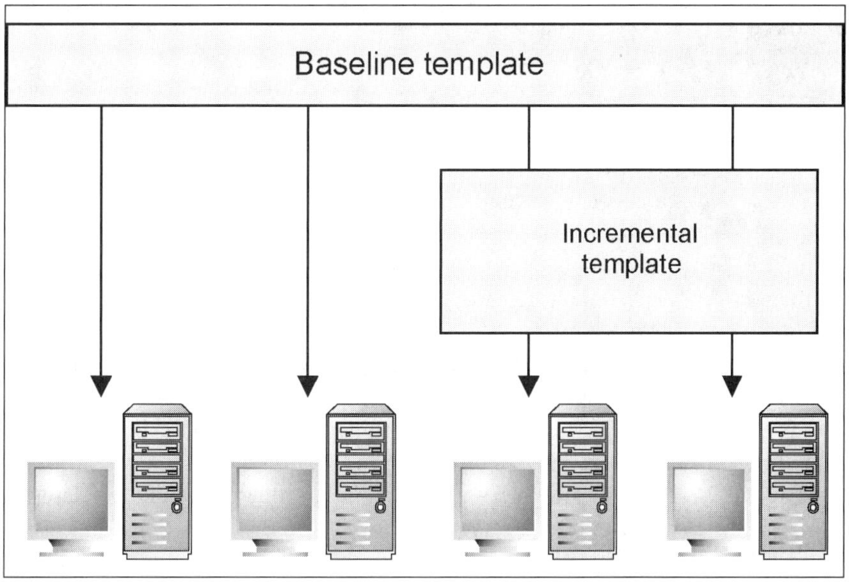

Figure 10-7 The Security for Print Spooler dialog box

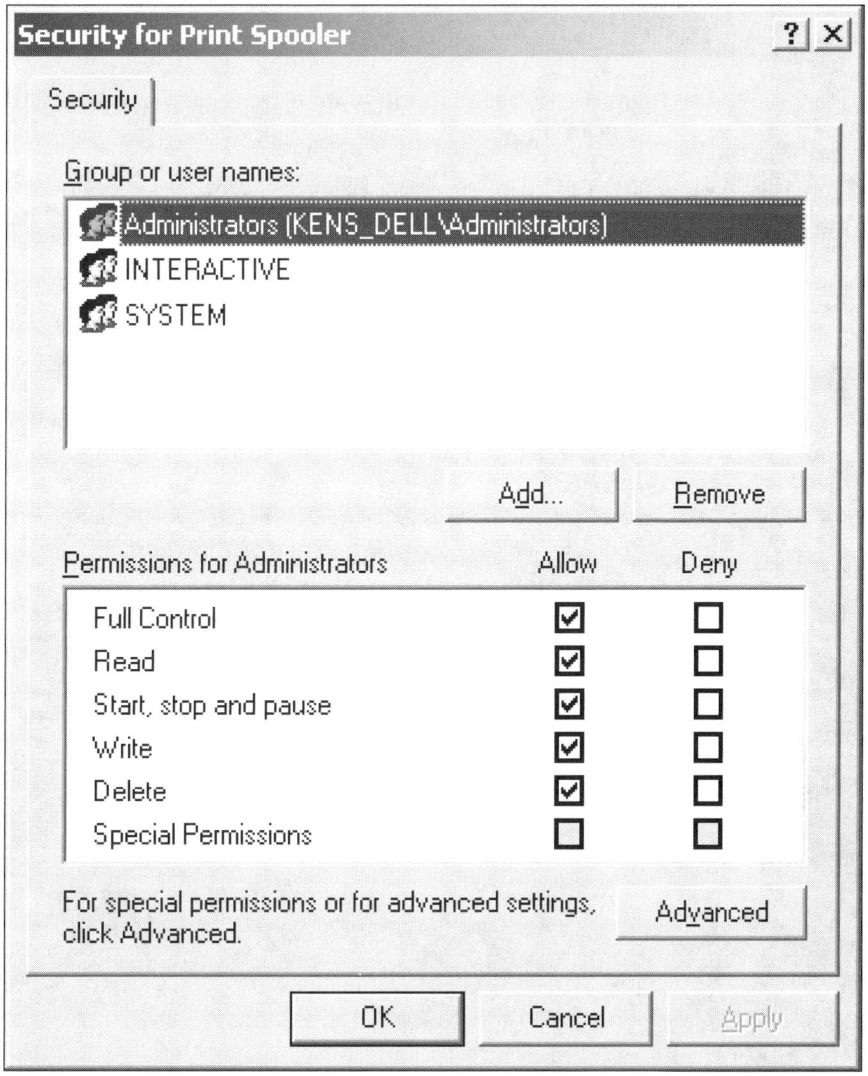

project 10.3

Using Incremental Security Templates *(cont'd)*

exam objective

Design security for servers that have specific roles. Roles include domain controllers, network infrastructure server, file server, IIS server, terminal server, and POP3 mail server. Create a plan to modify baseline security templates according to role.

project steps

18. Right-click **Security Configuration and Analysis** and click **Open Database**.
19. The **Open database** dialog box appears. Name the database **PrintServerTest** and click **Open**.
20. The **Import Template** dialog box opens. Select **baseline.inf** and click **Open**. The **Console Root** window reappears.
21. Right-click **Security Configuration and Analysis** in the right pane of the **Console Root** window and choose **Analyze Computer Now**.
22. The **Perform Analysis** dialog box opens. Accept the default path for the error log and click **OK**.
23. Double-click **System Services** in the left pane of the **Console Root** window and check the status of the **Print Spooler** service. It should say **Automatic** in the **Startup** column and **Configured** in the **Permission** column **(Figure 10-8)**.
24. Right-click **Security Configuration and Analysis** in the right pane of the **Console Root** window and choose **Configure Computer Now**.
25. The **Configure System** dialog box opens. Accept the default path for the error log and click **OK**.
26. Right-click **Security Configuration and Analysis** and choose **Analyze Computer Now**.
27. The **Perform Analysis** dialog box appears. Accept the default path for the error log and click **OK**.
28. Expand **Security Configuration and Analysis** in the left pane, click **System Services**, and check the status of the **Print Spooler** service. It should say **OK** in both the **Startup** and **Permission** columns.
29. Double-click **Print Spooler** and verify that the startup mode is **Disabled**, and then click **Cancel**.
30. Right-click **Security Configuration and Analysis** and choose **Import Template**.
31. The **Import Template** dialog box opens. Select **PrintServer.inf** and click **Open**.
32. Right-click **Security Configuration and Analysis** and choose **Analyze Computer Now**.
33. Accept the default path for error log file in the **Perform Analysis** dialog box and click the **OK** button.
34. Select **System Services** and note that, because the Print Spooler service in the database is different than that defined on the computer, **Investigate** now appears in both the **Startup** and **Permission** columns **(Figure 10-9)**.
35. Double-click **Print Spooler**. Notice that the database setting is as defined in the incremental template.
36. Close the MMC console. Do not save changes.

Figure 10-8 The new settings for the Print Spooler service in the Print Server template

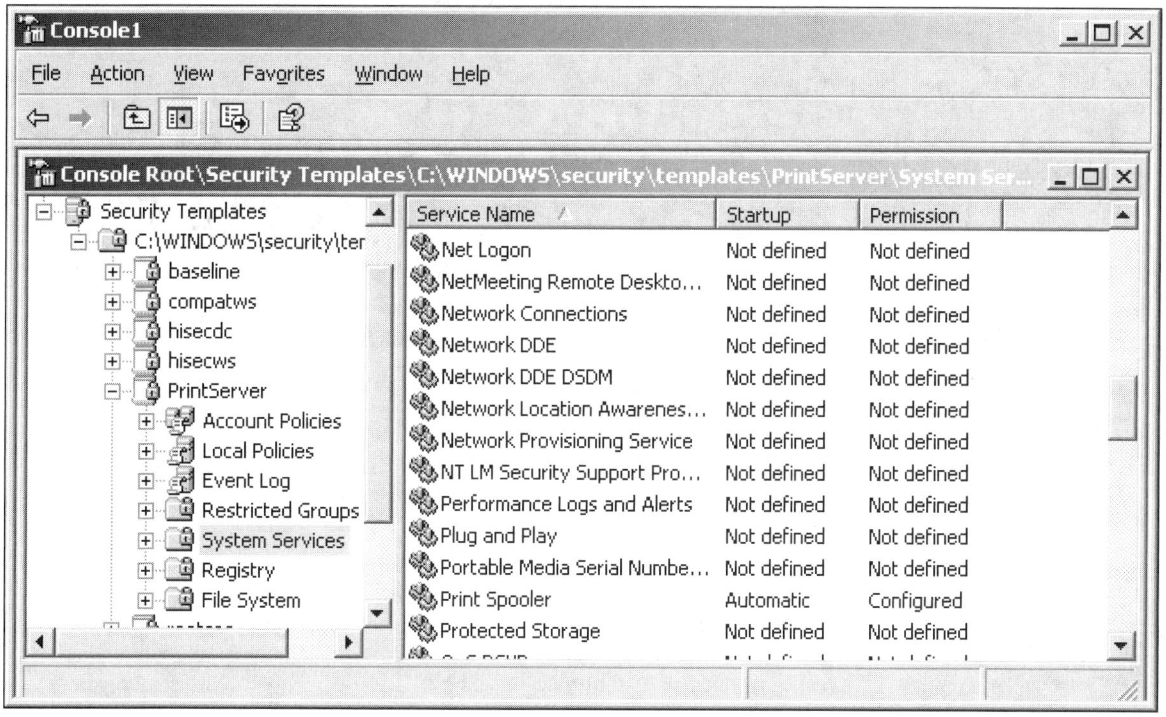

Figure 10-9 The Investigate message alerts you that settings defined on the computer do not match those in the template

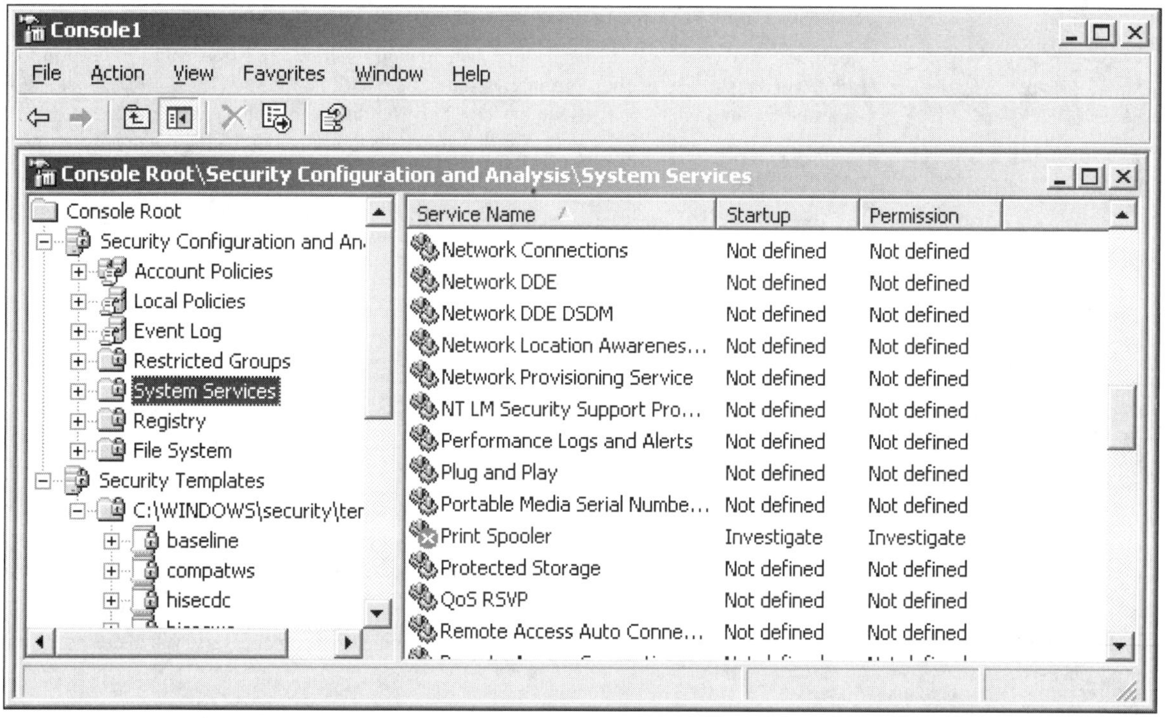

LESSON

11 Designing an Access Control Strategy for Data

Data security design is a careful balancing act involving several security components. It requires an understanding of how security is applied, evaluated, and tracked.

Resource access permissions are determined by access control entries (ACEs) in an object's system access control list (SACL) and discretionary access control list (DACL). Unless explicitly blocked, permissions assigned to a parent object (such as a folder) are inherited by any child objects (such as files). Permissions can be assigned to a user account or to a group. Permissions assigned to a group are automatically inherited by the group's members.

The order in which ACEs are evaluated can be significant. Denied permissions are evaluated first and take precedence over allowed permissions. Explicitly assigned permissions are evaluated before inherited permissions.

With file and folder permissions, both local access and share permissions must be considered. Local access permissions are supported by the NTFS file system only. When both local and share permissions apply to a user, the most restrictive permission set applies.

Encryption is another way of protecting data. If you wish to use Microsoft's Encrypting File System (EFS), you must format the computer's hard disk with the NTFS file system because EFS is not supported by the FAT32 or FAT file system. You should disable encryption until you have determined how it will be supported. A key part of supporting encryption is identifying data recovery agents (DRAs) who can decrypt data that was encrypted by another user.

A critical part of any security design is the backup and restore strategy. A backup is often your only chance of recovering data after a catastrophic failure. You must include:

- The data to be backed up
- The backup schedule
- Offsite secure storage of critical backups
- Recovery policies and procedures

A security design typically includes delegation of rights necessary to perform administrative tasks to selected users and groups. This makes it possible for identified users or groups to assist with limited administrative tasks, such as creating and managing users and groups in a single organizational unit (OU).

Auditing is an important part of protecting both network resources and Active Directory objects. You should limit auditing to critical resources or to provide a trail when you suspect unauthorized activity. An audit policy can include the activities to audit as well as whether auditing tracks successful events, failed events, or both.

Avoid making your data security design more complicated than necessary. When designing data security, whenever possible:

- Avoid changing permissions at the drive root.
- Assign permissions to folders instead of files.
- Assign permissions to groups instead of individual users.
- Use predefined groups when appropriate.
- Limit the number of DRAs.
- Set and adhere to backup schedules.
- Avoid delegating more rights or permissions than required.
- Implement auditing on an as-needed basis.

Scenario

You are working with the newly created Security department to create a data security design for Ready-Biz. You are working with key personnel to identify mission-critical data and data access requirements.

One potential concern is that some department managers want a level of administrative control over their users. There is also a need to identify some technical personnel to handle specific administrative tasks after normal hours and on weekends.

Lesson 11 Designing an Access Control Strategy for Data

Project	Exam 70-298 Objective
11.1 Designing Permission Structures	**Design an access control strategy for directory services.** Design the appropriate group strategy for accessing resources. Design a permission structure for directory service objects. **Design an access control strategy for the registry**. Design a permission structure for Registry objects. **Design an access control strategy for files and folders**. Design a permission structure for files and folders.
11.2 Understanding Delegation Strategies	**Design an access control strategy for directory services**. Create a delegation strategy.
11.3 Analyzing Auditing Requirements	**Design an access control strategy for directory services**. Analyze auditing requirements. **Design an access control strategy for files and folders**. Analyze auditing requirements. **Design an access control strategy for the registry**. Analyze auditing requirements.
11.4 Securing Backup and Recovery Strategies	**Design an access control strategy for directory services**. Design security for a backup and recovery strategy.
11.5 Designing a Strategy for Encrypting and Decrypting Files and Folders	**Design an access control strategy for directory services**. Design a strategy for the encryption and decryption of files and folders.

General Requirements

To complete the projects in this lesson, you will need administrative rights on a Windows XP Professional or Windows Server 2003 computer with at least one disk partition formatted with NTFS. You may also find it helpful to refer to Lesson 11 in your Prentice Hall Certification Series Exam 70-298 textbook for additional information about the topics covered by the projects in this lesson.

project 11.1

Designing Permissions Structures

exam objective

Design an access control strategy for directory services. Design the appropriate group strategy for accessing resources. Design a permission structure for directory service objects.

Design an access control strategy for the registry. Design a permission structure for registry objects.

Design an access control strategy for files and folders. Design a permission structure for files and folders.

overview

The Security department will have direct responsibility for company-wide shared servers. Departmental managers will be responsible for identifying departmental access requirements, which will be implemented by technical personnel or delegated users. Security will be managed through local access security **(Figure 11-1)** and share security **(Figure 11-2)**.

You are responsible for providing guidelines for data access security best practices. You need to provide both general guidelines and sample detailed instructions for common security scenarios.

learning objective

After completing this project, you will understand guidelines for applying data access permissions.

specific requirements

None

estimated completion time

10 minutes

project steps

1. Prepare a short document justifying the use of NTFS on all disk volumes hosting shared folders.
2. Prepare a short document explaining the relationship between local and shared access security.
3. As one of your specific examples, identify how to configure security to meet access requirements for an Accounts Payable server **(Figure 11-3)** as follows:
   - Users must log on locally to modify data.
   - Local and network users can view data or run reports based on server data.

Figure 11-1 NTFS local access security

- Folder permissions
  - Read
  - Write
  - List Folder Contents
  - Read & Execute
  - Modify
  - Full Control
- File permissions
  - Read
  - Write
  - Read & Execute
  - Modify
  - Full Control

Figure 11-2 Shared access security

- Share permissions
  - Read
  - Change
  - Full Control

Figure 11-3 Accounts Payable server access requirements

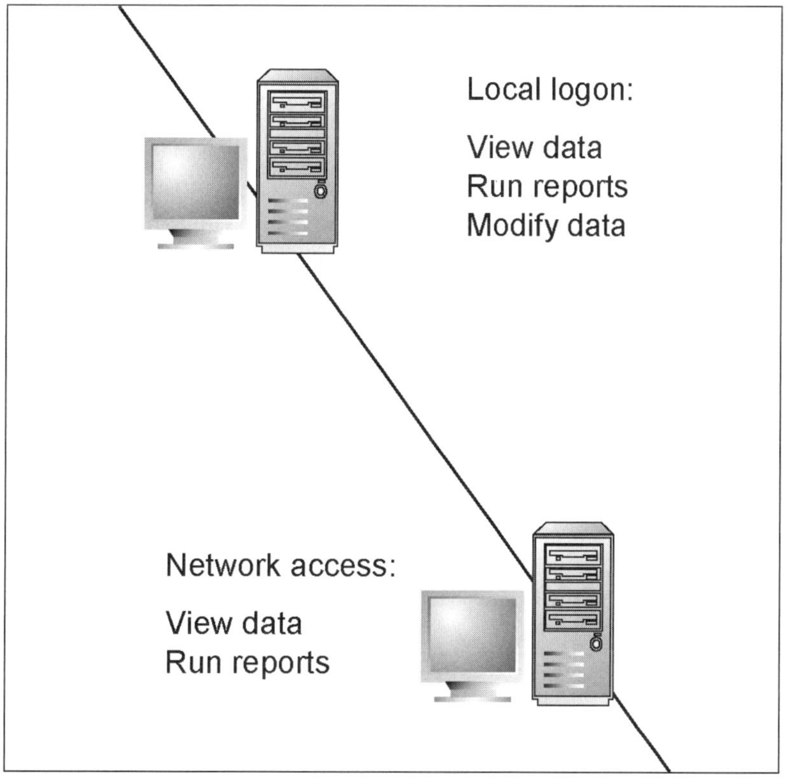

project 11.2

Understanding Delegation Strategies

exam objective

Design an access control strategy for directory services. Create a delegation strategy.

overview

You have already prepared general delegation guidelines, shown in **Figure 11-4**. You are working with departmental managers to help them identify the specific delegation requirements.

Each department is responsible for managing user and group accounts specific to that department. Departmental managers will identify the personnel responsible for managing users and groups.

learning objective

After completing this project, you will understand requirements for designing a delegation strategy.

specific requirements

None

estimated completion time

10 minutes

project steps

1. Why is it better to delegate control through a security group than to individual users?
2. Describe the Active Directory OU structure best suited to the stated delegation requirements.
3. The OU structure of the United States division warehouse department is shown in **Figure 11-5**. Each OU contains user and group accounts. How should you configure delegation to allow three select users to manage all warehouse user and group accounts?
4. The security department wants to ensure that both administrative permissions and access to administrative tools are limited. How can you limit access to administrative tools?

Figure 11-4 General delegation guidelines

- Use predefined groups when possible.
- Delegate control at the highest possible level.
- Delegate control to security groups.
- Limit delegation by object type.
- Limit delegation, when possible, by attribute.
- Provide custom management consoles.

Figure 11-5 OU structure for the warehouse

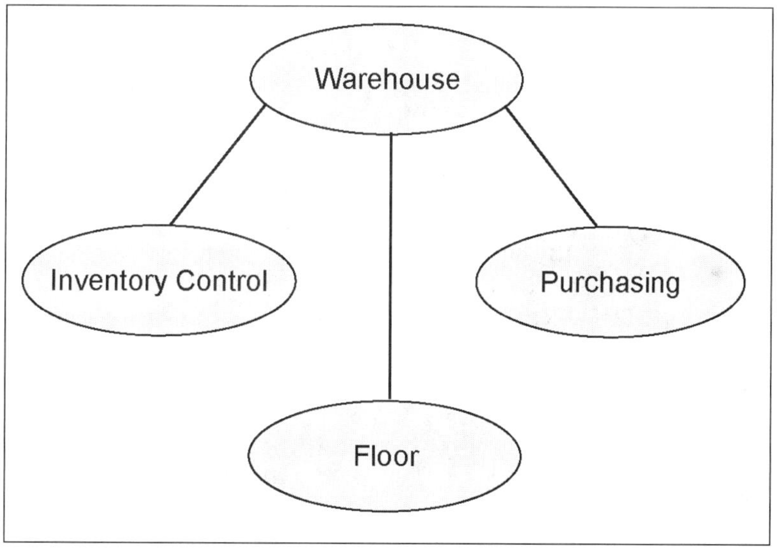

project 11.3

Analyzing Auditing Requirements

exam objective

Design an access control strategy for directory services. Analyze auditing requirements.
Design an access control strategy for files and folders. Analyze auditing requirements.
Design an access control strategy for the registry. Analyze auditing requirements.

overview

Ready-Biz has not used auditing in the past. You have proposed gradually introducing auditing of key resources and critical activities. This includes educating decision makers about available audit policies **(Table 11-1)**, the policies most appropriate to the company's requirements, and general justification for investing the time and effort necessary to implement auditing **(Figure 11-6)**.

learning objective

After completing this project, you will understand justifications and requirements for implementing auditing.

specific requirements

None

estimated completion time

15 minutes

project steps

1. Prepare a short report justifying the need to implement domain-wide audit policies.
2. In each of the following situations, describe how auditing should be configured to meet the auditing requirements.
    - There should a record made of any changes made to user or group accounts by users delegated to manage departmental OUs.
    - All unsuccessful attempts to access all financial records should be logged.
    - Any attempts to log on to the domain or locally to an individual client should be recorded.
    - There is a need for an historical record of any changes made to audit policy after it is first established.

Table 11-1 Audit policies

Policy	Description
Audit account logon events	Records events associated with an account being authenticated by the security database. If a user logs on locally to a machine, the event is recorded in the machine's event log. If the user authenticates by logging onto the domain, it is recorded in the domain controller's event log. Logging this type of information provides the security identifier of the account that failed or succeeded and also the name of the computer, its domain or workgroup, and the type of logon attempt.
Audit account management	Records the creation, modification, or deletion of a user account or group. This includes renaming a user account, disabling it, or changing or resetting the password.
Audit directory service access	Records an event when a user accesses an Active Directory object.
Audit logon events	Records events associated with a user logging on or off of a local computer. It also records events when a user attempts a network connection to a remote computer. The event is recorded in the security event log of the computer where the logon attempt occurs. If the user connects to a remote computer, a logon event is recorded in the security event log on the remote computer.
Audit object access	Records events when a user accesses a file, folder, or printer.
Audit policy change	Records events when security options are changed. Examples might include changing a user right, modifying an audit policy, or modifying account policies.
Audit privilege use	Records events associated with a user exercising user rights. For example, Melissa changes the system time or takes ownership of William's files.
Audit process tracking	Records actions performed by applications. Used by programmers for debugging application issues.
Audit system events	Records events that affect the security logs, or situations where the computer has been shut down or restarted. These are considered to be events that impact Windows Server 2003 security.

Figure 11-6 Advantages of auditing

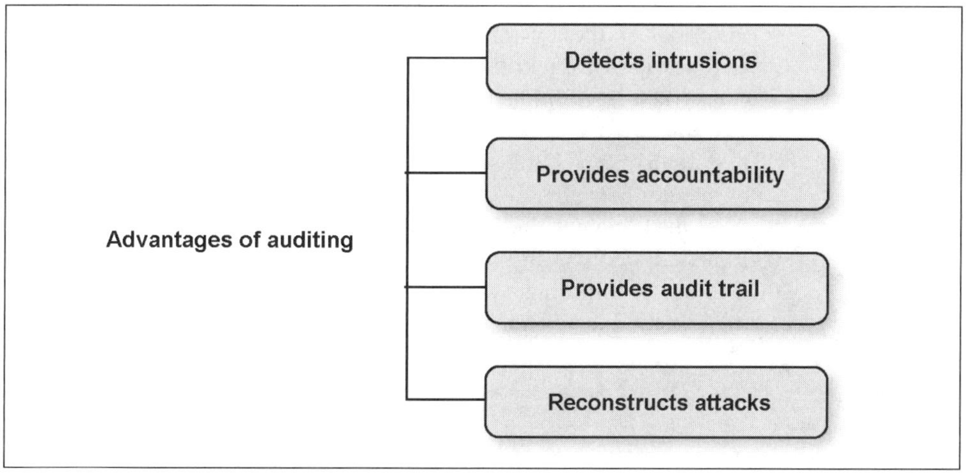

project 11.4

Securing Backup and Recovery Strategies

exam objective

Design an access strategy for directory services. Design security for a backup and recovery strategy.

overview

Most critical resources are being backed up on a relatively consistent basis, but Ready-Biz does not have company-wide policy for data backups and disaster recovery. You need to work with network administrators to develop backup and restore strategies that can then be applied to other divisions **(Figure 11-7)**.

One major concern is that administrators have not placed any emphasis on backing up System State data on any network servers. You need to provide specific steps for backing up System State data.

learning objective

After completing this project, you will know how to design a backup strategy.

specific requirements

You need access to a computer running Windows XP Professional or Windows Server 2003. You must be logged on as a user with sufficient permission to back up System State data.

estimated completion time

10+ minutes. System State backup times vary between computers.

project steps

You will step through the procedures for backing up System State data.

1. Open **Windows Explorer** and create a folder named **BackupTest** in the root of the **C:** drive.
2. Click **Start,** point to **All Programs**, point to **Accessories**, point to **System Tools**, and then click **Backup**.
3. The **Backup and Restore Wizard** appears. Choose **Advanced Mode**.
4. The **Backup Utility** window appears **(Figure 11-8)**. Click the **Backup** tab.
5. First, select the **System State** check box under **My Computer** and then select **C:\BackupTest\Backup.bkf** as the Backup media or file name.
6. Click **Start Backup**.
7. The **Backup Job Information** dialog box opens. Click **Start Backup**. As noted above, the length of time for the backup to complete will vary depending on the number and size of the files being backed up.
8. After the backup is finished, click **Close**.
9. Exit the **Backup** utility.
10. Answer the following questions:
    (a) What backup media types are compatible with offsite storage?
    (b) Why should backup copies be stored offsite?

Figure 11-7 Backup/restore strategies

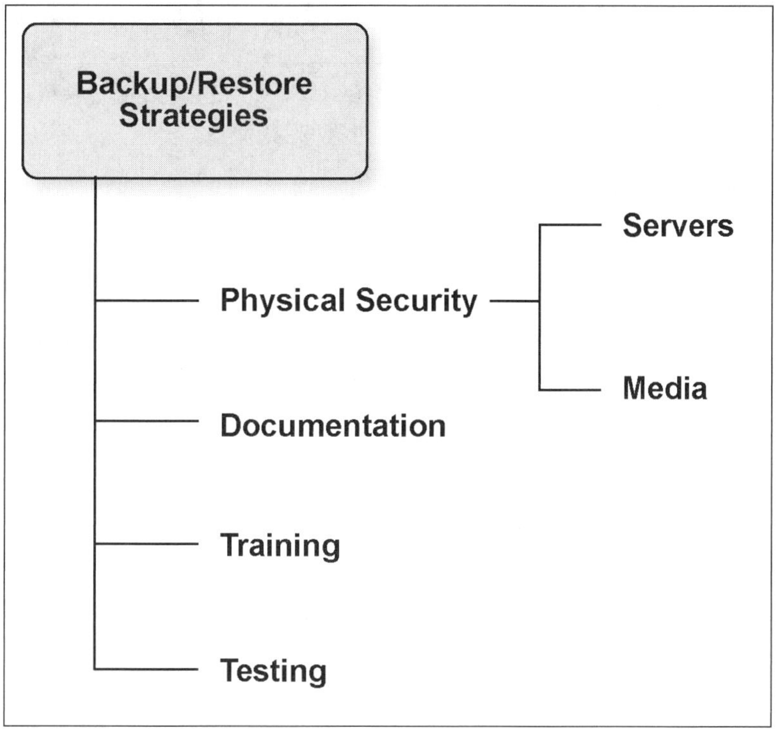

Figure 11-8 The Backup Utility window

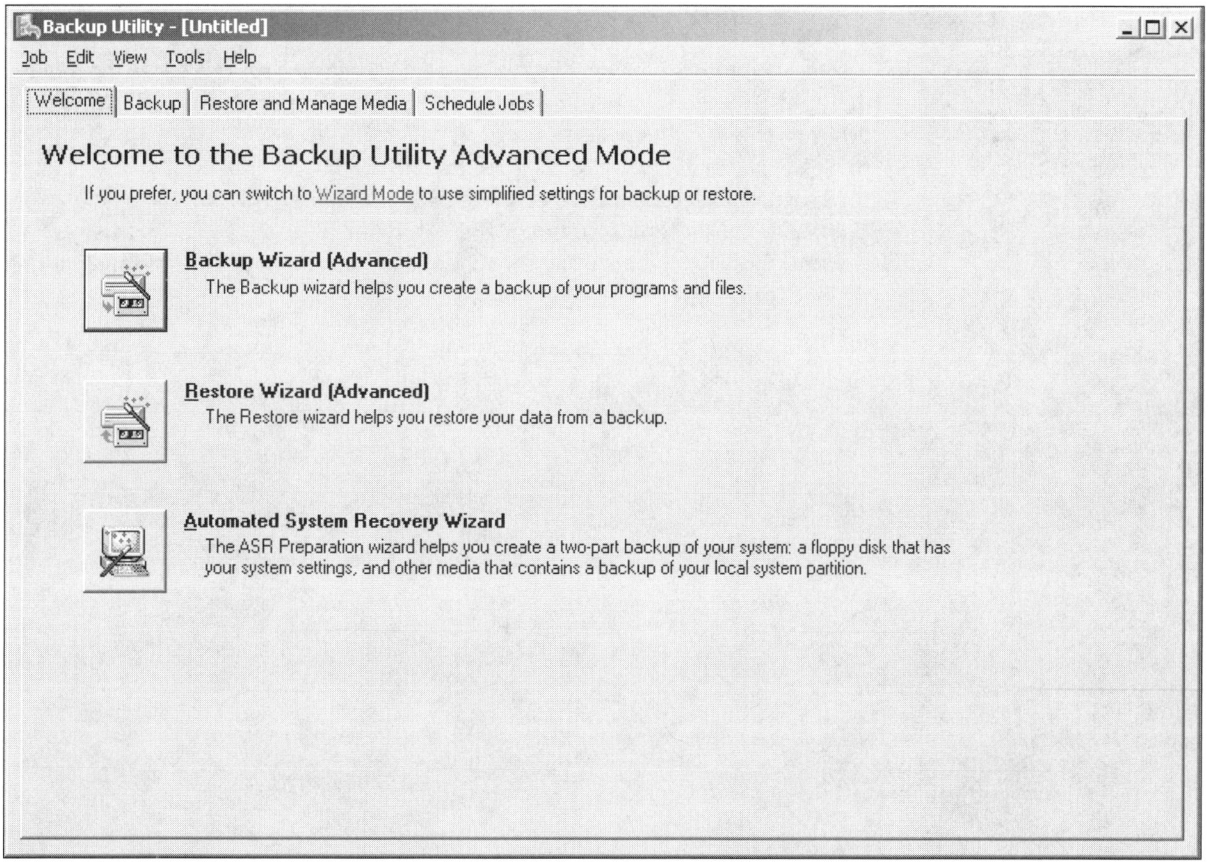

project 11.5

Designing a Strategy for Encrypting and Decrypting Files and Folders

exam objective

Design an access control strategy for directory services. Design a strategy for the encryption and decryption of files and folders.

overview

You are reviewing the security design requirements for mobile users. Local user accounts on mobile computers will be password-protected. Business-confidential data will be protected through NTFS right assignments and data-encrypted. DRAs will be configured through domain policy **(Figure 11-9)**.

You want to make sure that mobile users understand both how portable computers are configured and why. This includes an understanding of the encryption process **(Figure 11-10)**.

learning objective

After completing this project, you will know how to configure data encryption.

specific requirements

You need access to a computer running Windows XP or Windows Server 2003. The C: drive must be formatted as NTFS.

estimated completion time

10 minutes

project steps

1. Open **Windows Explorer** and create a folder named **Secure Files** in the root of drive **C:**.
2. Right-click the **Secure Files** folder and open its **Properties** dialog box.
3. On the **General** tab, click **Advanced**.
4. Select **Encrypt contents to secure data**.
5. Save the changes to the folder's properties.
6. Prepare a short description of the role of DRAs and why they are critical to managing encryption. Write the report from the standpoint of information important to mobile users.

Figure 11-9 EFS policy recovery agents in default domain policy

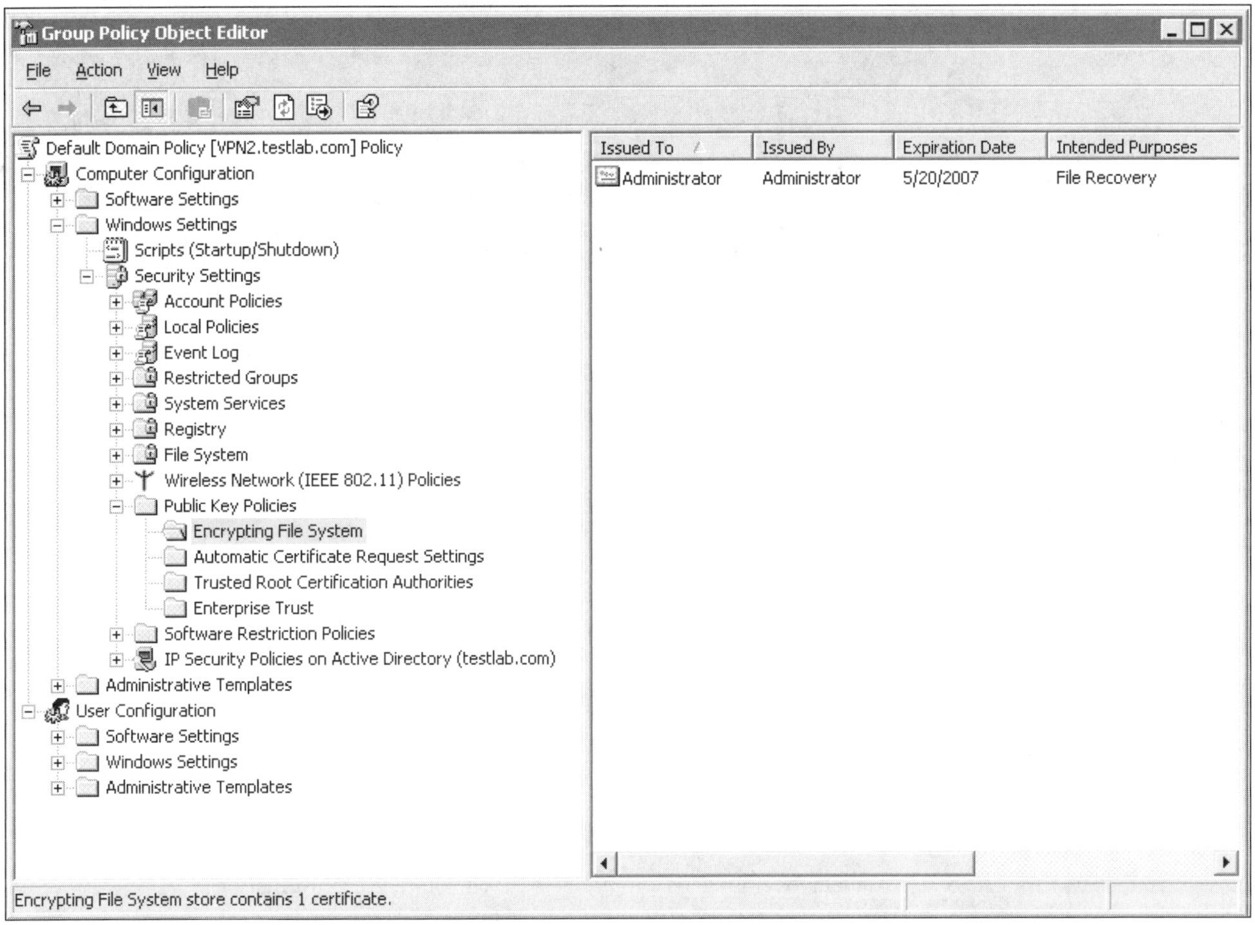

Figure 11-10 EFS encryption process

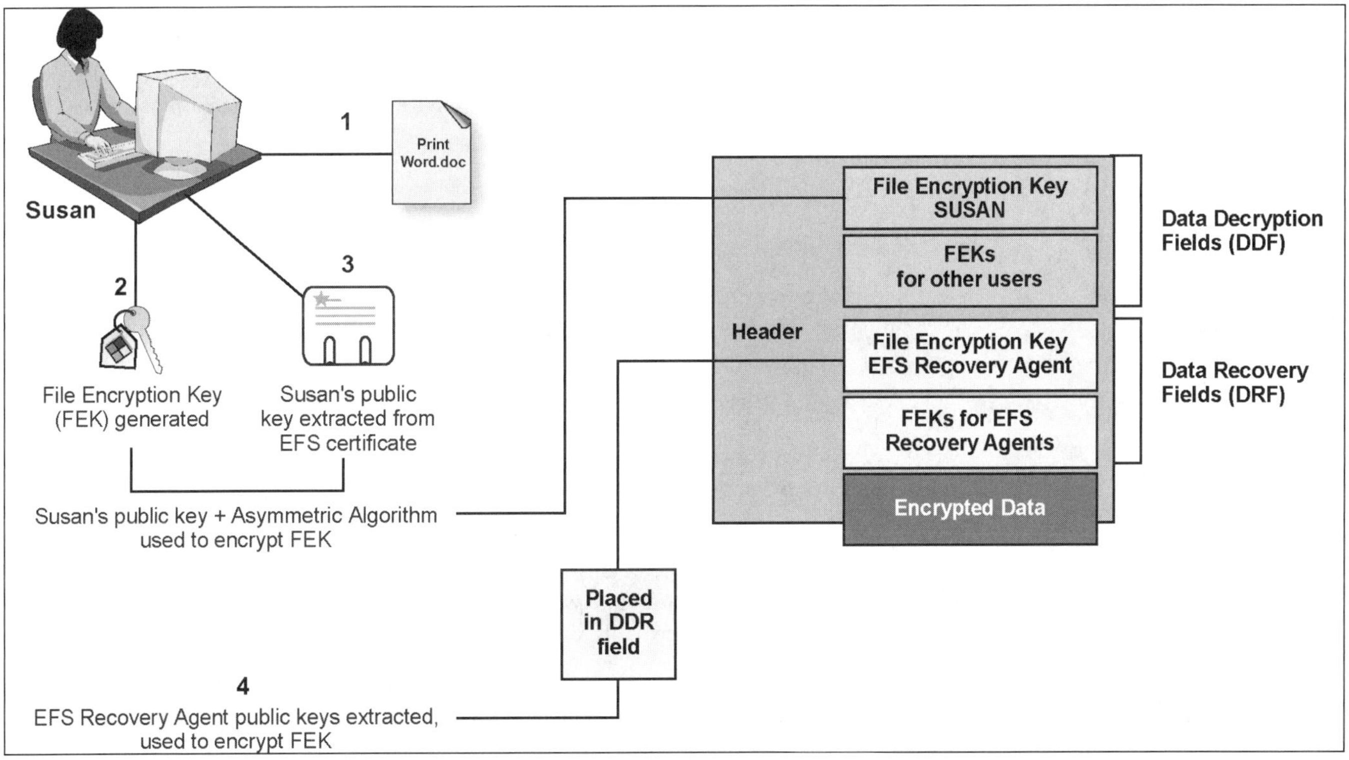

LESSON

12 Creating the Physical Design for Client Infrastructure Security

Authentication is the process of validating that a user is who he or she claims to be. An effective authentication strategy can help to ensure that you know who is accessing your network, can authorize those users to access only specific resources, and can audit their actions on the network. Designing an authentication strategy requires that you consider the following:

- Which client operating systems will issue requests for authentication?
- How will users connect to the network? Options include:
  - Local area network
  - Dial-up
  - VPN
  - Wireless
- Which operating system or database will store user information?
- What credentials will you accept as proof of user identity?

After you have answered these questions, you can begin to design an authentication strategy that will adhere to your company's security policy and provide assurance that you know who is accessing resources on your network.

One decision you will need to make is which authentication protocols to use on the local area network (LAN). Windows Server 2003 supports the following authentication protocols:

- LAN Manager
- NTLM
- NTLM v2
- Kerberos

Kerberos is the most secure authentication protocol, but can only be used between when authenticating Windows 2000 (and later) domain members in a Windows 2000 (or later) domain or when authenticating Unix and Linux clients. NTLM v2 is a good solution when supporting legacy Microsoft clients, such as Windows 98 and Windows NT 4, because Active Directory client software is available to allow these operating systems to authenticate using NTLM v2. NTLM is used with older Windows NT operating systems. LAN Manager should be used only when supporting pre-Windows 98 computers.

If you need to support remote access or wireless clients, you must make a number of other decisions. The Routing and Remote Access Service (RRAS) allows you to define policies that limit which users can connect remotely and during which hours. Additional constraints, such as the number from which they are calling or the media used to connect, can also be established.

If you need to support multiple remote access or virtual private network (VPN) servers or if you need to support authenticating switches or wireless access points, you will probably want to implement a Remote Authentication Dial-In User Service (RADIUS) server to centralize remote access policies. Microsoft's implementation of RADIUS is the Internet Authentication Service (IAS).

Scenario

You are working with a team made of up individuals from each of the offices in the United States to design an authentication strategy. You must consider authentication requirements for the following types of users:

- Users in the Chicago office
- Users in the regional offices
- Users who connect through dial-up
- Users who connect through a VPN
- Users who connect through a wireless access point

As you'll recall, the Chicago office hosts the forest root domain. A child domain is implemented at each site. All domain controllers are running Windows Server 2003. The following client operating systems must be supported:

- Windows 98
- Windows NT 4 Workstation
- Windows 2000 Professional
- Windows XP Professional
- Linux

The Linux computers were added when Ready-Biz recently acquired a small marketing company. That company's personnel include users who were physically relocated to the Philadelphia office and a small number of telecommuters. All Linux computers are in a Kerberos realm in the Philadelphia office. The telecommuters have laptop computers running Linux. These users connect to the network through a VPN.

The company would like to set up wireless access points in the Chicago office. These access points will be used primarily by employees visiting from the regional offices and by telecommuters when they are in the office. The wireless network in the Chicago office will be a trial run. If it can be implemented securely, wireless networks will be set up in other offices.

Lesson 12 Creating the Physical Design for Client Infrastructure Security

Project	Exam 70-298 Objective
12.1 Analyzing Authentication Requirements	**Design a client authentication strategy**. Analyze authentication requirements. Establish account and password security requirements.
12.2 Understanding Remote Access Policies	**Design a client authentication strategy**. Design a security strategy for client remote access. Design access to internal resources. Design remote access policies.
12.3 Designing Authentication/Accounting Strategies Using Internet Authentication Service	**Design a client authentication strategy**. Design an authentication provider and accounting strategy for remote network access.

General Requirements

There are no special requirements for this lesson. However, you may find it helpful to refer to Lesson 12 in your Prentice Hall Certification Series Exam 70-298 textbook for additional information about the topics covered by the projects in this lesson.

project 12.1

Analyzing Authentication Requirements

exam objective

Design a client authentication strategy. Analyze authentication requirements. Establish account and password security requirements.

overview

You are analyzing the company's security requirements and determining the most secure authentication protocols to use and the type of credentials to accept. As you'll recall, you must consider company requirements, compatibility issues with legacy operating systems and non-Microsoft operating systems, and application requirements **(Figure 12-1)**.

You must identify the protocols that can be used for local authentication and remote access authentication. You must also evaluate whether usernames and passwords are the best credentials to use or if the company should migrate to two-factor authentication using smart cards.

learning objective

After completing this project, you will know how to select appropriate authentication protocols and identify the requirements for smart card authentication.

specific requirements

None

estimated completion time

10 minutes

project steps

1. Your company would like to limit LAN authentication to NTLM v2 and Kerberos. What change or changes will need to be made to the client operating systems?
2. Which remote access authentication protocols must be enabled on the remote access and VPN servers to support all clients?
3. Which remote access authentication protocols should be enabled on the Windows XP Professional computers that will connect to a VPN server?
4. Which user account passwords must be stored in reversibly encrypted format?
5. What is the best way to allow Linux clients to be authenticated by domain controllers?

Figure 12-1 Analyzing authentication requirements

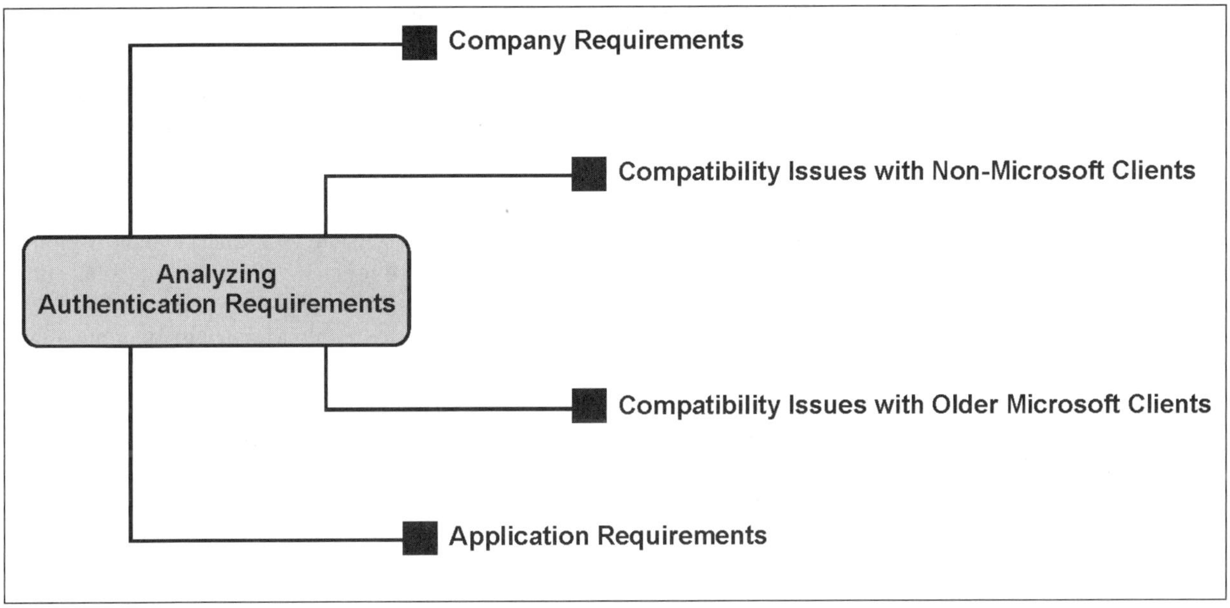

project 12.2

Understanding Remote Access Policies

exam objective

Design a client authentication strategy. Design a security strategy for client remote access. Design access to internal resources. Design remote access policies.

overview

You are designing a security policy for users who will connect to servers in the Chicago office through remote access and VPN. You must determine the appropriate user account dial-up settings and remote access policy conditions. As you'll recall, permission is granted or denied based on a combination of the user account dial-up settings, the remote access policy conditions, and whether the client can accept the remote access profile settings. The flow chart shown in **Figure 12-2** can help you determine whether a user will be allowed or denied access under specific conditions.

The remote access and VPN clients need to be able to access several file servers on the network. You want to assign an IP configuration, including the address of the DNS server using DHCP.

The remote access security requirements are as follows:

- Only members of the Sales, Telecommuters, Executives, and Domain Admins groups should be allowed to connect to the network through a VPN or dial-up connection.
- Telecommuters are limited to connecting through a VPN connection.
- The Telecommuters and Sales groups can connect only Monday through Saturday from 7 A.M. to 8 P.M.
- Members of the Executives and Domain Admins groups need to be able to connect 24x7.
- Members of the Sales and Executives groups need to be able to supply a call-back number when connecting through a dial-up connection.
- Temporary employees should not be allowed to connect to the network through a VPN or remote access connection.

learning objective

After completing this project, you will know how to design a remote access and VPN solution to meet specific requirements.

specific requirements

None

estimated completion time

15 minutes

project steps

1. How many remote access policies will you implement?
2. Create a document outlining the conditions that will be implemented in each policy.
3. How will you configure the user accounts of members of these groups?
4. How will you prevent members of the Temporary Employees group from connecting through a remote access or VPN connection?
5. What steps must you take to enable users who connect to access file servers on the internal network?

Figure 12-2 Policy application flow chart

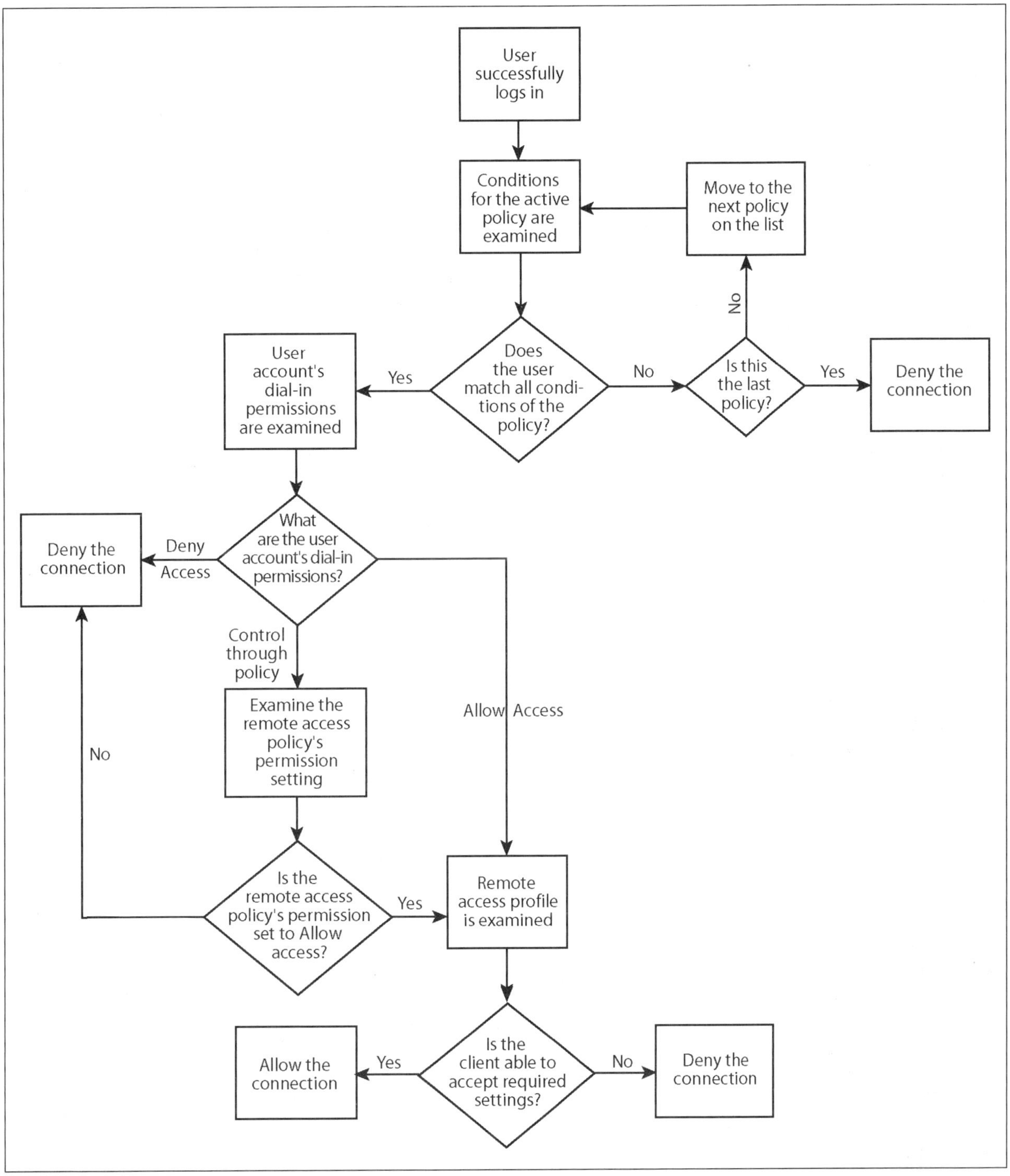

project 12.3

Designing Authentication/Accounting Strategies using Internet Authentication Service

exam objective

Design a client authentication strategy. Design an authentication provider and accounting strategy for remote network access.

overview

You must develop a strategy to centralize authentication policy management for remote access, VPN access, and wireless access at the Chicago office. To meet usage requirements, you will need 2 remote access servers, 3 VPN servers, and 14 wireless access points. You have decided to use RADIUS to centralize remote access policies. As you'll recall, RADIUS clients send a RADIUS message to the RADIUS server, as shown in **Figure 12-3**.

Previously, you learned that placement of servers on a network is an important part of ensuring they are secure. When designing network security for the Chicago office, you implemented two firewalls: one between the Internet and a screened subnet, and the other between the screened subnet and the private network, as shown in **Figure 12-4**. A wireless network has also been integrated with the internal network. The domain controllers are located on the internal network. You must determine where to place the VPN servers and the RADIUS server (or servers) to provide the most secure solution. Keep in mind the following considerations:

- The VPN server passes the user's credentials to the RADIUS server.
- The RADIUS server passes the user's credentials to the domain controller.
- The VPN server receives encrypted data packets from the users.
- Company policy requires that data packets be examined by a firewall before being allowed into the internal network.

learning objective

After completing this project, you will know how to design a remote access solution that includes RADIUS servers.

specific requirements

None

estimated completion time

10 minutes

project steps

1. On which network segment will you place the RADIUS server(s)?
2. On which network segment will you place the VPN servers?
3. How many RADIUS clients will the Chicago office have?
4. How can you provide fault tolerance for the RADIUS server(s)?
5. How can you allow users in the Executives group to be subject to different remote access policies when connected to the wireless network than when connected over a dial-up or VPN connection?

Figure 12-3 RADIUS server

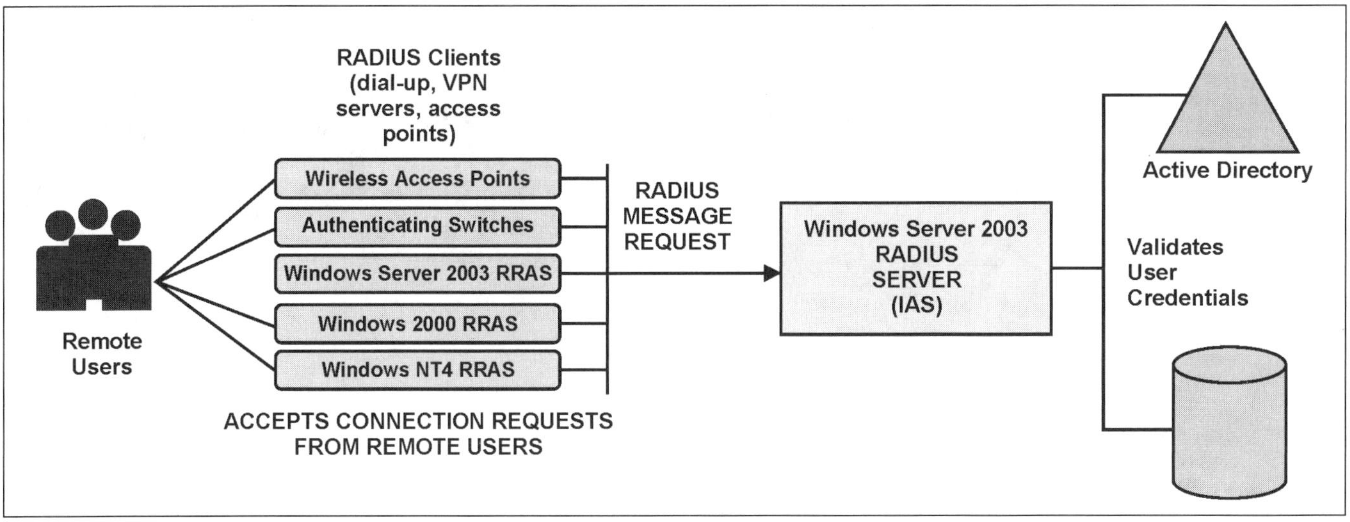

Figure 12-4 Chicago network segmentation

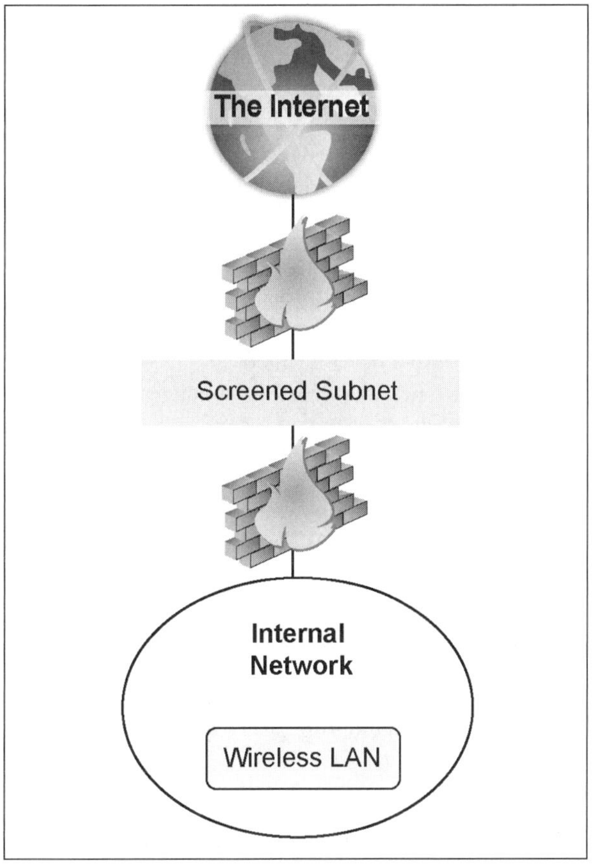

LESSON 13

Securing Client Computers

A common flaw in security design is that insufficient attention is paid to client computer requirements. Unsecured or improperly secured client systems can be an open back door into your network.

A good starting point for securing client computers is careful consideration of the security life cycle. The basic life cycle is defined as:

- Installation: Install using an image, or from known good, uncompromised installation media and apply available security updates as part of the installation process.
- Baseline configuration: Apply an appropriate baseline security template, as described in Lesson 10.
- Role-specific security: Identify the role or roles to be performed by the client and apply appropriate incremental security.
- Security updates: Apply incremental security updates and service packs as available, typically managed through the Windows Automatic Updates service.
- Decommissioning: Take the client out of service when no longer needed, clearing the computer of any secure or sensitive information.

You need to understand the settings applied through the predefined administrative security templates, as well as what you can and cannot do through security policy settings. You must keep in mind that an important part of client security management is user management. It is possible to defeat well-defined security policies through inappropriate user rights and permissions. Whenever possible, manage users through rights and permissions assigned to groups. Avoid granting membership to local groups with elevated permissions, such as the Administrators and Power Users groups.

The most efficient way to manage client security is through an Active Directory domain environment. Active Directory lets you:

- Organize client computers by OU
- Organize client computers by group
- Apply baseline and incremental security templates through Group Policy

Care must be taken in designing your organizational unit (OU) structure to meet your needs. Common designs including basing the structure by operating system, by strategic role, or by geographic location. Avoid the temptation to make the structure more complicated than is required by your security needs.

Make use of predefined administrative templates whenever possible and apply incremental changes as necessary. Key considerations include:

- Set strong password policy to prevent unauthorized logon and access.
- Set software restriction policies to limit allowed software and prevent use of unauthorized software.
- Use the Certificate Rule to control software execution through certificates from a trusted source.

- Use the Hash Rule to control access by creating a hash of the application executable or other required file.
- Use the Internet Zone Rule to control software downloaded and installed from the Internet.
- Use the Path Rule to restrict access to file and directory paths.
- Use auditing to monitor logon and account management activities.
- Encrypt account management data to and from domain controllers.
- Limit local machine access (local logon rather than domain logon) and remote access to administrators only.
- Use EFS to protect locally-stored sensitive information.

It is important to test security templates, including default templates provided with the operating system, before their use in a production environment.

Scenario

Up to now, the security plan has focused on securing servers, network communications, Internet access, and user logon and access. You now need to work on designing client security.

Client security will be rolled out on a per-domain basis to allow for testing. The current plan is to implement client security plans in one of the smaller United States division domains first so that problems can be resolved before applying the plans to the larger domains. This time, Chicago will be one of the last domains to which the changes are applied.

Lesson 13 Securing Client Computers

Project	*Exam 70-298 Objective*
13.1. Designing Strategies for Hardening Client Computers	**Design a strategy for securing client computers.** Considerations include desktop and portable computers. Design a strategy for hardening client operating systems.
13.2. Designing Strategies for Restricting User Access to Operating System Features	**Design a strategy for securing client computers.** Considerations include desktop and portable computers. Design a strategy for restricting user access to operating system features.

General Requirements

There are no special requirements for this lesson. You may find it helpful to refer to Lesson 13 in your Prentice Hall Certification Series Exam 70-298 textbook for additional information about the topics covered by the projects in this lesson.

project 13.1

Designing Strategies for Hardening Client Computers

exam objective

Design a strategy for securing client computers. Considerations include desktop and portable computers. Design a strategy for hardening client operating systems.

overview

You need to start designing client system security based on the computer security life cycle (**Figure 13-1**). You will need to identify baselines, administrative templates, and incremental custom templates. This includes developing rule-based guidelines for security applications (**Figure 13-2**).

It may be necessary to develop a new OU structure to meet the security design requirements. The OU structure is currently organized around departments, grouping departmental users and computers.

learning objective

After completing this project, you will understand guidelines for security client computers.

specific requirements

None

estimated completion time

15 minutes

project steps

1. Prepare a description as background material for the security design, describing the importance of including client computers in the security design.
2. As part of your guidelines on setting security policy, explain the difference between setting an option as Not Configured, Enabled, or Disabled, and the impact on previously applied policies.
3. You are provided with sample OU structures as guidelines for restructuring the company's domains (**Figure 13-3**). Design two potential OU structures:
   - Retain the departmental structure, but support applying group policy by operating system.
   - Separate computers from the departmental structure and support applying group policy by client role.
4. Based on your structures designed in Step 3, which would be easiest to manage?

Figure 13-1 Life cycle of computer security

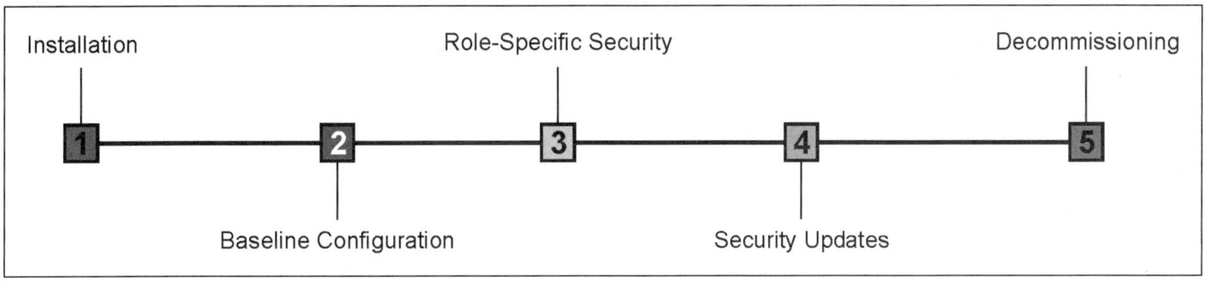

Figure 13-2 The order in which rules are applied

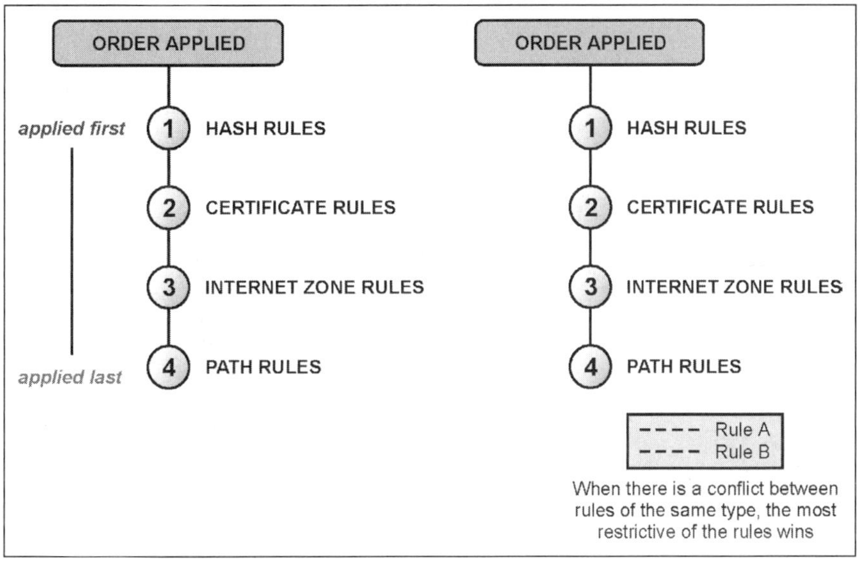

Figure 13-3 OU structural examples

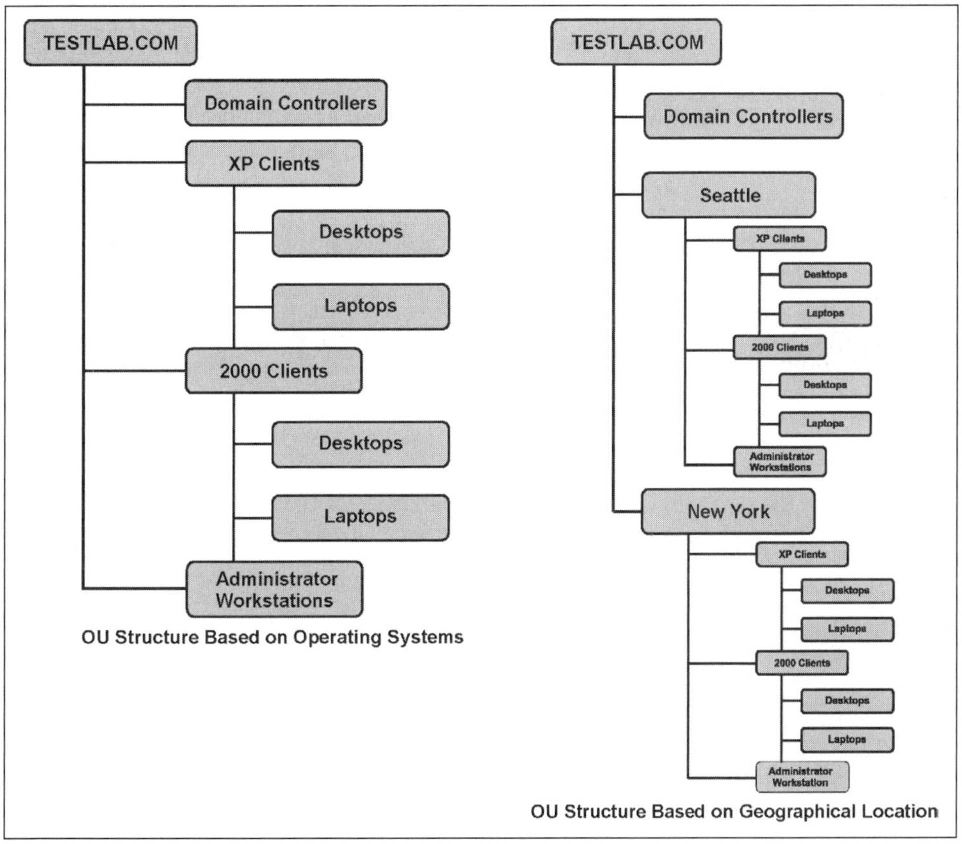

project 13.2

Designing Strategies for Restricting User Access to Operating System Features

exam objective

Design a strategy for securing client computers. Considerations include desktop and portable computers. Design a strategy for restricting user access to operating system features.

overview

You want to avoid introducing potential backdoors into the security system because of inappropriate user access. You are reviewing security policies in detail and have asked all personnel in the security department to review the online Windows XP Security Guide (**Figure 13-4**).

The following concerns must be addressed:

- Limit access to operating system files.
- Limit access to the Registry.
- Do not allow users to add or remove software.
- Do not allow users to add or remove printers or other peripherals.

Users will be allowed to change desktop appearance. A user will also be able to shut down the client computer to which he or she is logged on.

learning objective

After completing this project, you will know how to develop guidelines for restricting user access to operating system features.

specific requirements

None, but you will need to apply concepts learned in earlier lessons to complete this project.

estimated completion time

10 minutes

project steps

1. Some users must run an application that will not run with the permissions assigned to the Users group. Possible solutions are adding the domain user account to the computer's Power Users group or applying the Compatws.inf template. Compare these solution options.
2. How does the principle of least privilege (**Figure 13-5**) apply in this situation? Refer to Lesson 5, if necessary.

Figure 13-4 Windows XP Security Guide

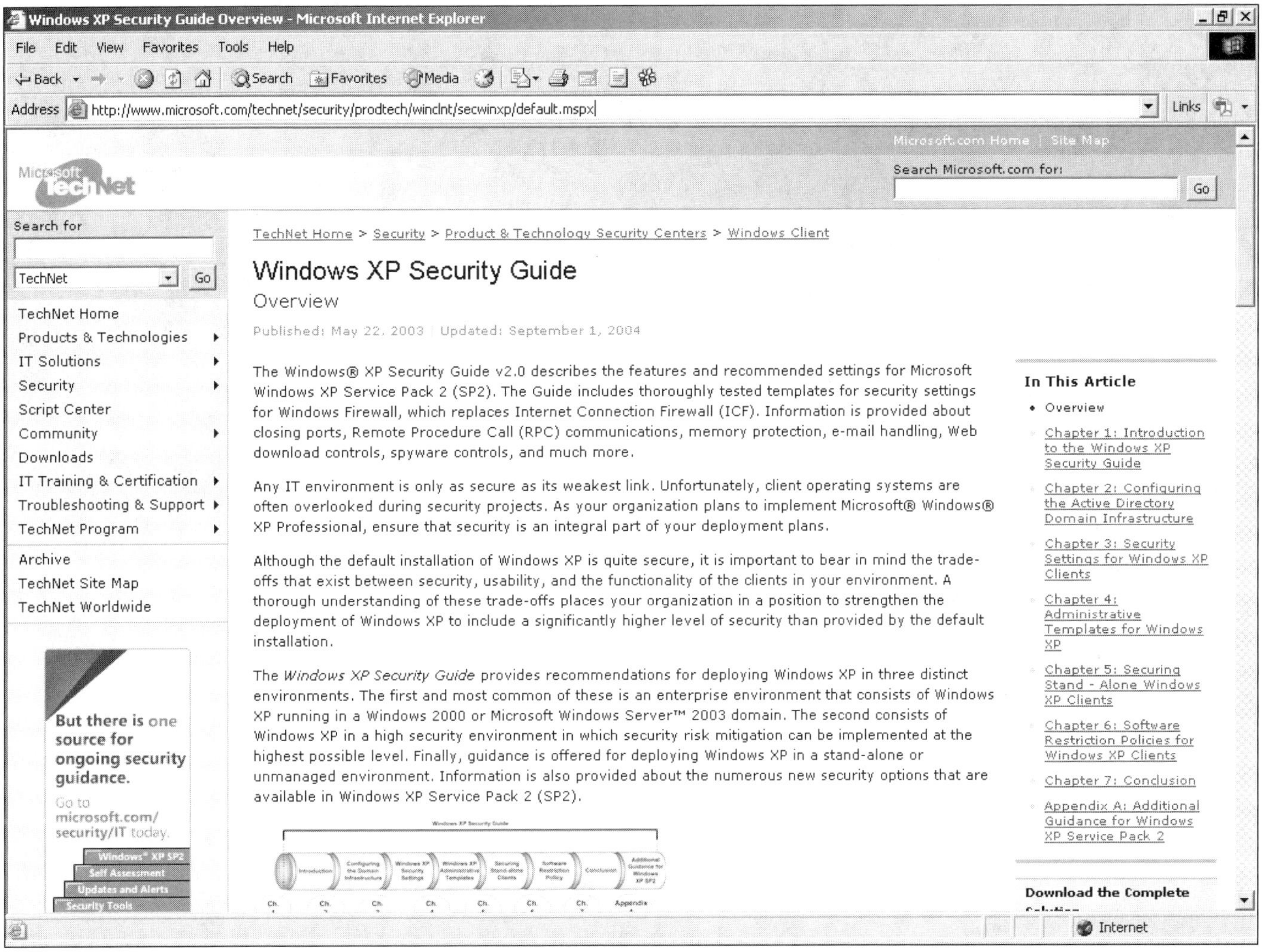

Figure 13-5 Principle of least privilege

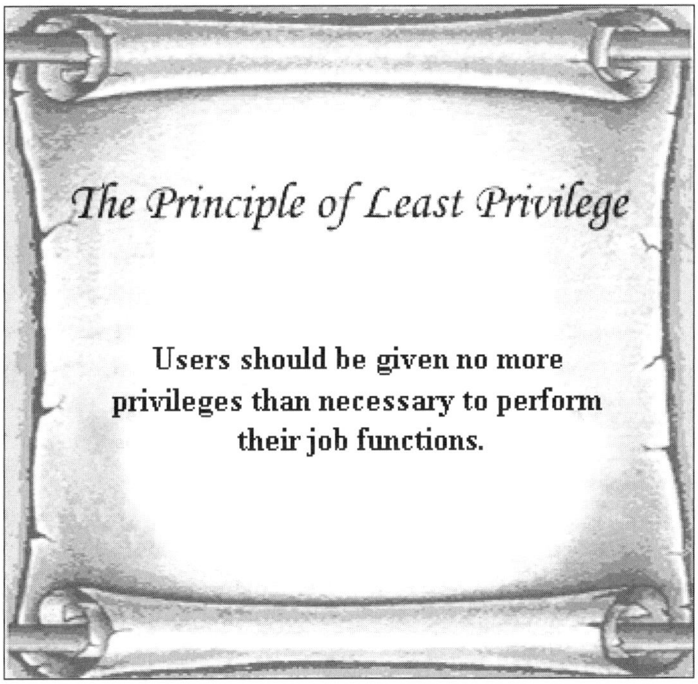

LESSON 14

Securing Internet Information Services (IIS)

A Web server is often the most public server on a company's network. Companies use Web servers to create a point of presence on the Internet, to conduct e-commerce, and to offer customers information and support. However, a Web server can also store confidential information and be used internally for a variety of purposes. When designing security for a company's Web server, you need to keep in mind the company's goal, the type of information it will store, who need to access stored information, the privacy requirements of information transferred over the network, and whether that information will be transferred across the company's intranet only or across the Internet as well.

Depending on the type of content a Web server provides, you may need to enable various services. All Web servers require the World Wide Web Publishing service and the HTTP SSL service. Web servers might also require services, such as Internet Server Application Programming Interfaces (ISAPI), Active Server Pages (ASP), or ASP.NET, to provide dynamic content or access to databases. They might also offer additional services, such as File Transfer Protocol (FTP), Simple Mail Transfer Protocol (SMTP), or Network News Transfer Protocol (NNTP). It is essential that you enable only the required services on a Web server. Enabling unnecessary services increases the attack surface of the server.

In addition to identifying the services that must be enabled, you must plan for ongoing updates and monitoring. Various update strategies are available, including FTP, Web-based Distributed Authoring and Versioning (WebDAV), and FrontPage Server Extensions. IIS 6.0 also offers several monitoring options, including customizable W3C Extended Log File format, Microsoft IIS Log File format, NCSA Common Log File format, ODBC-compliant database logging, and centralized binary logging. You must choose the logging method that is the most suitable to your requirements.

Finally, you must select an authentication method. Although most public Web sites allow anonymous access, intranet Web sites and those to which a subscription is required must authenticate a user's identity. IIS 6.0 supports authentication using Integrated Windows Authentication, Digest Authentication, Advanced Digest Authentication, Basic Authentication, and authentication using client certificates.

Scenario

You are working with a team made of up individuals from each of the offices in the United States. The team has been asked to design security for an intranet Web site that will perform inventory tracking of materials used in the manufacturing process. It will also serve as a repository for specifications for current and upcoming products.

All users in the company need to be able to access specific resources on the Web server. The inventory-tracking application is under development and will use ASP.NET. HTML versions of the specifications will be created using Front Page. In-process specifications will be available for upload or download only to product engineers. The initial proposal calls for uploads and downloads using FTP.

You must design security to meet the company's requirement. You will configure a test computer for testing your security assumptions and the Web content.

Lesson 14 Securing Internet Information Services (IIS)

Project	Exam 70-298 Objective
14.1 Securing Web Sites by Enabling the Minimum Services	**Design security for Internet Information Services (IIS).** Design security for Web sites that have different technical requirements by enabling only the minimum required services. Design an IIS baseline that is based on business requirements.
14.2 Designing a Content Management Strategy for IIS	**Design security for Internet Information Services (IIS).** Design a content management strategy for updating an IIS server.
14.3 Designing a Monitoring Strategy for IIS	**Design security for Internet Information Services (IIS).** Design a monitoring strategy for IIS.
14.4 Designing User Authentication for a Web Site	**Design security for Internet Information Services (IIS).** **Design user authentication for Internet Information Services (IIS).** Design user authentication for a Web site by using IIS authentication. Design user authentication for a Web site by using certificates.

General Requirements

To complete the projects in this lesson, you will need administrative rights on a Windows Server 2003 computer. You may find it helpful to refer to Lesson 14 in the Prentice Hall Certification Series Exam 70-298 textbook for additional information about the topics covered by the projects in this lesson.

project 14.1

Securing Web Sites by Enabling the Minimum Services

exam objective

Design security for Internet Information Services (IIS). Design security for Web sites that have different technical requirements by enabling only the minimum required services. Design an IIS baseline that is based on business requirements.

overview

You must configure a Web server to use for testing. The server must have the necessary services enabled. Some of these services can be enabled automatically during setup (**Figure 14-1**). Others need to be enabled using the Services snap-in. Still others will need to be enabled using the Web Service Extensions node in Internet Information Services (IIS) Manager.

You will configure the server by adding the Application server role, and then by enabling additional required services.

learning objective

After completing this project, you will know how to configure a Web server to run the necessary services.

specific requirements

A Windows Server 2003 computer without IIS installed. You will also need access to the Windows Server 2003 installation files to complete the optional project steps.

estimated completion time

15 minutes

project steps

1. Identify the services that must be enabled to meet the stated requirements.
2. Which of these services are enabled using the Services utility?
3. Which of these services are enabled using IIS Manager?

Optional Project Steps

4. Click **Start**, point to **Administrative Tools**, and then click **Configure Your Server Wizard**.
5. Click **Next** to open the **Preliminary Steps** screen.
6. Click **Next** to open the **Server Role** screen.
7. Select **Application server (IIS, ASP.NET) (Figure 14-2)** and click **Next**.
8. The **Application Server Options** screen opens. Select the **Enable ASP.NET** check box **(Figure 14-3)** and click **Next**.
9. The **Summary of Selections** screen opens. Click Next to open the **Applying Selections** screen. The **Windows Components Wizard/Configuring the Components** screen opens. You will be prompted to insert the Windows Server 2003 installation CD-ROM. Insert the CD and click OK.
10. After IIS has been installed and configured, the Windows Component Wizard closes, and the final page of the Configure Your Server Wizard opens to tell you that **This Server is Now an Application Server**. Click **Finish** to close the wizard.
11. Click **Start**, point to **Administrative Tools**, and then click **Services**.
12. Record the Startup type for the following services:
    - HTTP SSL
    - IIS Admin Service
    - World Wide Web Publishing Service
13. Close the Services snap-in.

Figure 14-1 Services node in the Computer Management console

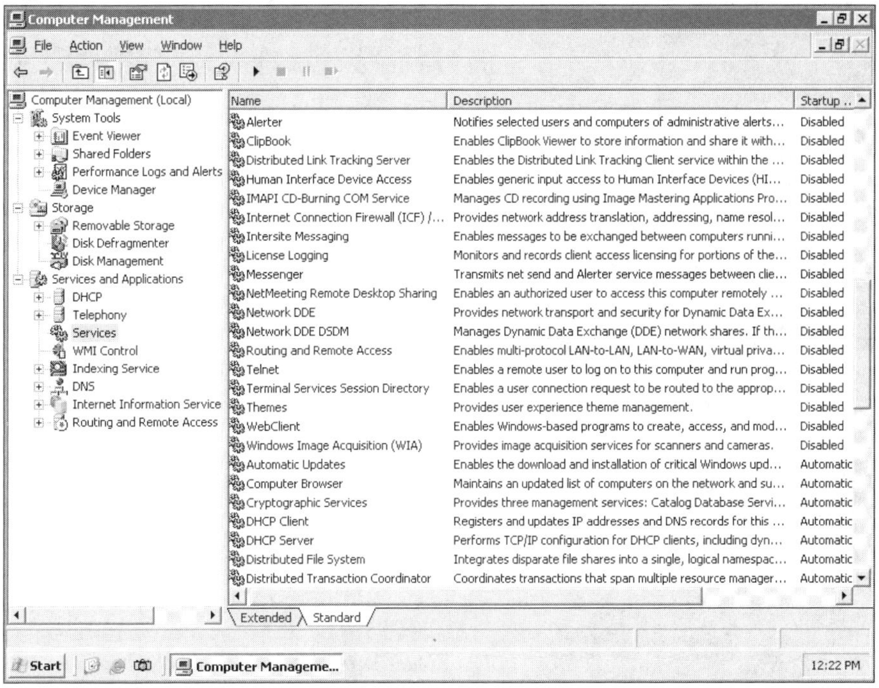

Figure 14-2 Configuring an Application server

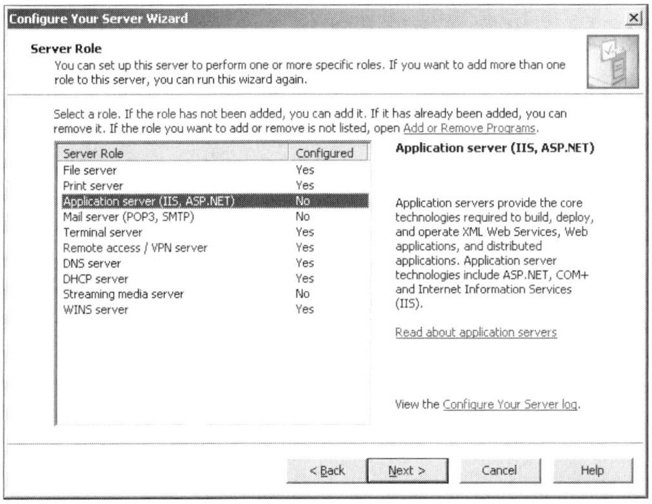

Figure 14-3 Enabling ASP.NET

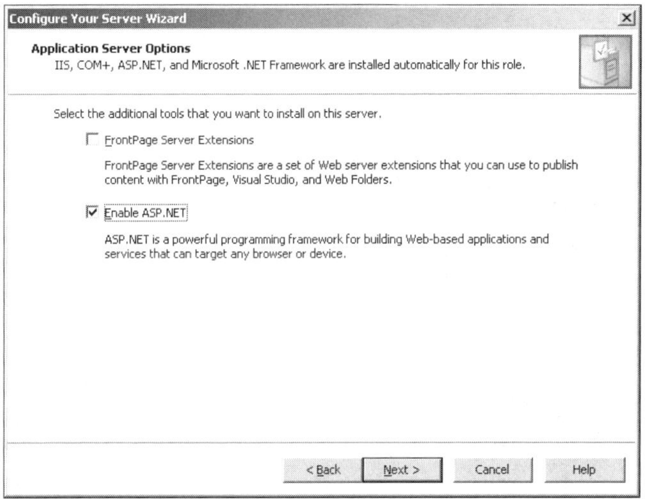

project 14.1

Securing Web Sites by Enabling the Minimum Services (cont'd)

exam objective

Design security for Internet Information Services (IIS). Design security for Web sites that have different technical requirements by enabling only the minimum required services. Design an IIS baseline that is based on business requirements.

project steps

14. Choose **Start**, point to **Administrative Tools**, and then click **Internet Information Services (IIS) Manager** to open the **Internet Information Services (IIS) Manager** snap-in.
15. Click your server to expand the node.
16. Click **Web Service Extensions (Figure 14-4)**.
17. Which service or services are allowed?
18. Close the Internet Information Services (IIS) Manager snap-in.
19. The FTP service is not installed by default when the application server role is installed. You will now install the FTP service. Click **Start**, click **Control Panel**, and then click **Add or Remove Programs**.
20. Click **Add/Remove Windows Components**.
21. Select **Application Server** and click **Details**.
22. Select **Internet Information Services (IIS)** and click **Details**.
23. Check **File Transfer Protocol (FTP Service)**. Click **OK**.
24. Click **OK**.
25. Click **Next**.
26. If prompted for the installation source files, browse to locate them and click **OK**.
27. Click **Finish**.
28. Close **the** Add or Remove Programs dialog box.

Figure 14-4 Web Service Extensions

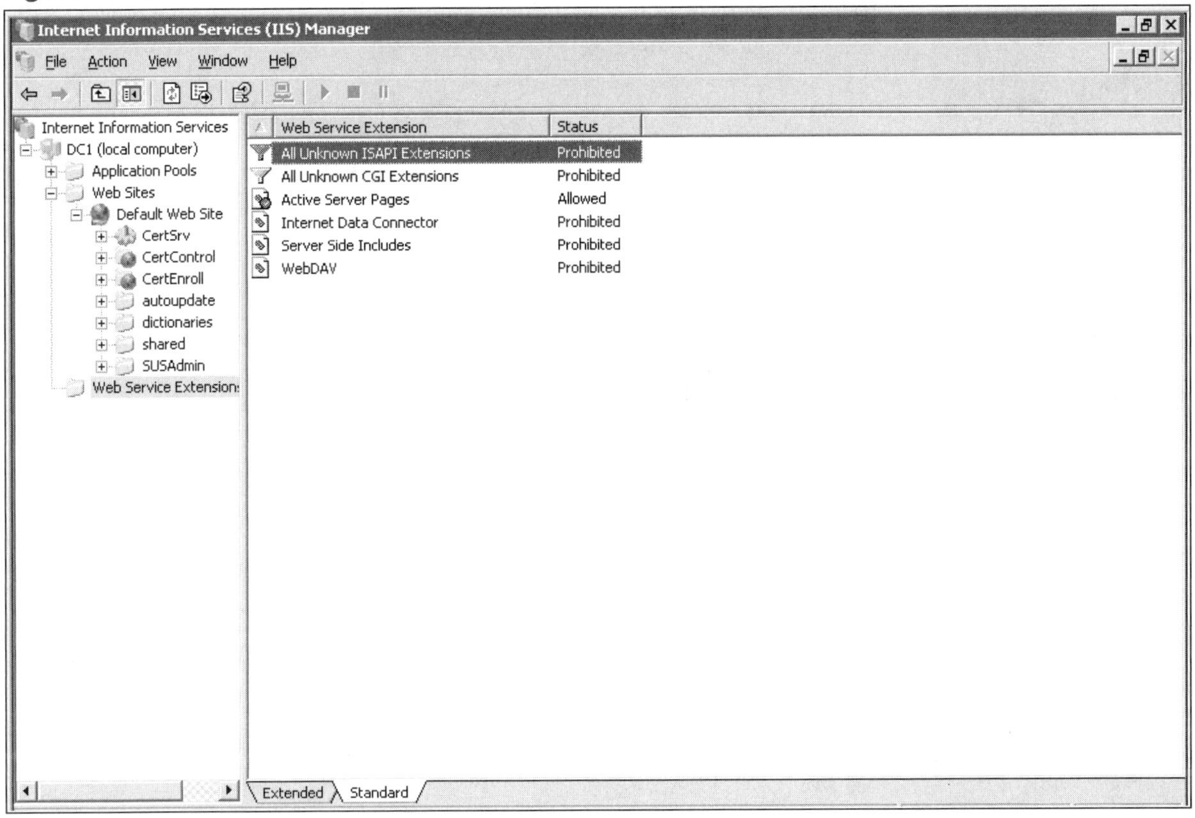

project 14.2

Designing a Content Management Strategy for IIS

exam objective

Design security for Internet Information Services (IIS). Design a content management strategy for updating an IIS server.

overview

You are evaluating the best way to update the content on the Web server. You must determine how the ASP.NET application files, Front Page files, and other documents will be uploaded to the Web server. The company has agreed that the application development manager will be responsible for all updates to the ASP.NET application. Several different users will be responsible for updating the specifications.

You must also secure administration of the Web server. All Web site management will be performed from a specific IP address. You can configure the Administration Web site to accept communication from one address only, as shown in **Figure 14-5**.

learning objective

After completing this project, you will know how to design a content deployment strategy to meet specific requirements.

specific requirements

IIS must be installed on a computer running Windows Server 2003 to complete the optional steps.

estimated completion time

10 minutes

project steps

1. What are the possible security problems with using FTP to update content on the Web server?
2. What are the client requirements for using WebDAV to update content on the Web server?
3. What are the benefits of using Front Page Server Extensions to update the HTML product specifications?

Optional Steps

4. Enable **WebDAV**.
5. Enable **Front Page Server Extensions**.

Figure 14-5 Selecting IP addresses that can administer Web site properties

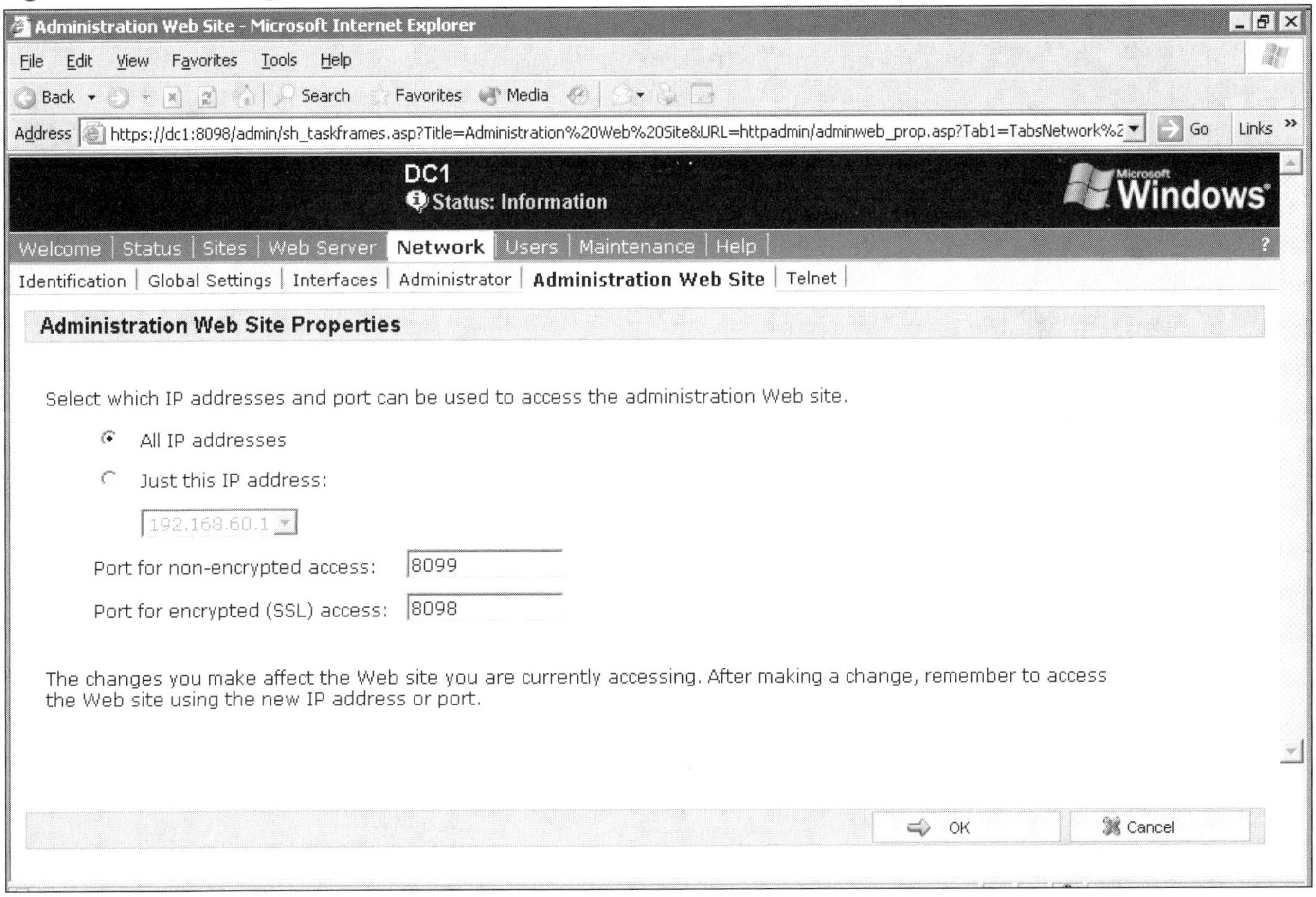

project 14.3

Designing a Monitoring Strategy for IIS

exam objective

Design security for Internet Information Services (IIS). Design a monitoring strategy for IIS.

overview

Another decision you must make is the type of logging to use on the Web site and the FTP site. The company requires that the following information be logged for all attempts to access the Web site and the FTP site:

- Date
- Time
- Client IP address
- User name
- Bytes sent
- Bytes received

A new log file for the Web site should be started daily. A new log file for the FTP site should be started when the file becomes 10 MB. Log formats are configured in a Web site's Properties dialog box or in an FTP site's Properties dialog box.

learning objective

After completing this project, you will know how to configure logging options.

specific requirements

To complete the optional project steps, a Windows Server 2003 computer with IIS and the FTP service installed.

estimated completion time

15 minutes

project steps

1. What logging format will you use for the Web site?
2. What logging format will you use for the FTP site?

Optional Project Steps

3. Open the **Internet Information Services (IIS) Manager** snap-in.
4. Click your server to expand the node.
5. Expand the **Web Sites** node **(Figure 14-6)**.
6. Right-click **Default Web Site** and click **Properties** to open the **Default Web Site Properties** dialog box.
7. Click the **Web Site** tab and verify that **W3C Extended Log File Format** is selected in the **Active log format** list box **(Figure 14-7)**.
8. Click **Properties** to open the **Logging Properties** dialog box.
9. Verify that **Daily** is selected in the **New log schedule** section **(Figure 14-8)**.
10. Click the **Advanced** tab and configure the extended logging options so that only the necessary information is logged.
11. Click **OK** to apply your selections and close the **Logging Properties** dialog box.
12. Click **OK** to close the **Default Web Site Properties** dialog box.
13. Expand the **FTP Sites** node.
14. Right-click **Default FTP Site** and click **Properties** to open the **Default FTP Site Properties** dialog box.
15. Which log formats are available?
16. Select W3C Extended Log File Format and click **Properties**.
17. Configure the General and Advanced properties as specified.
18. Close the Internet Information Services (IIS) Manager snap-in.

Figure 14-6 Web Sites node in the Internet Information Services (IIS) Manager snap-in

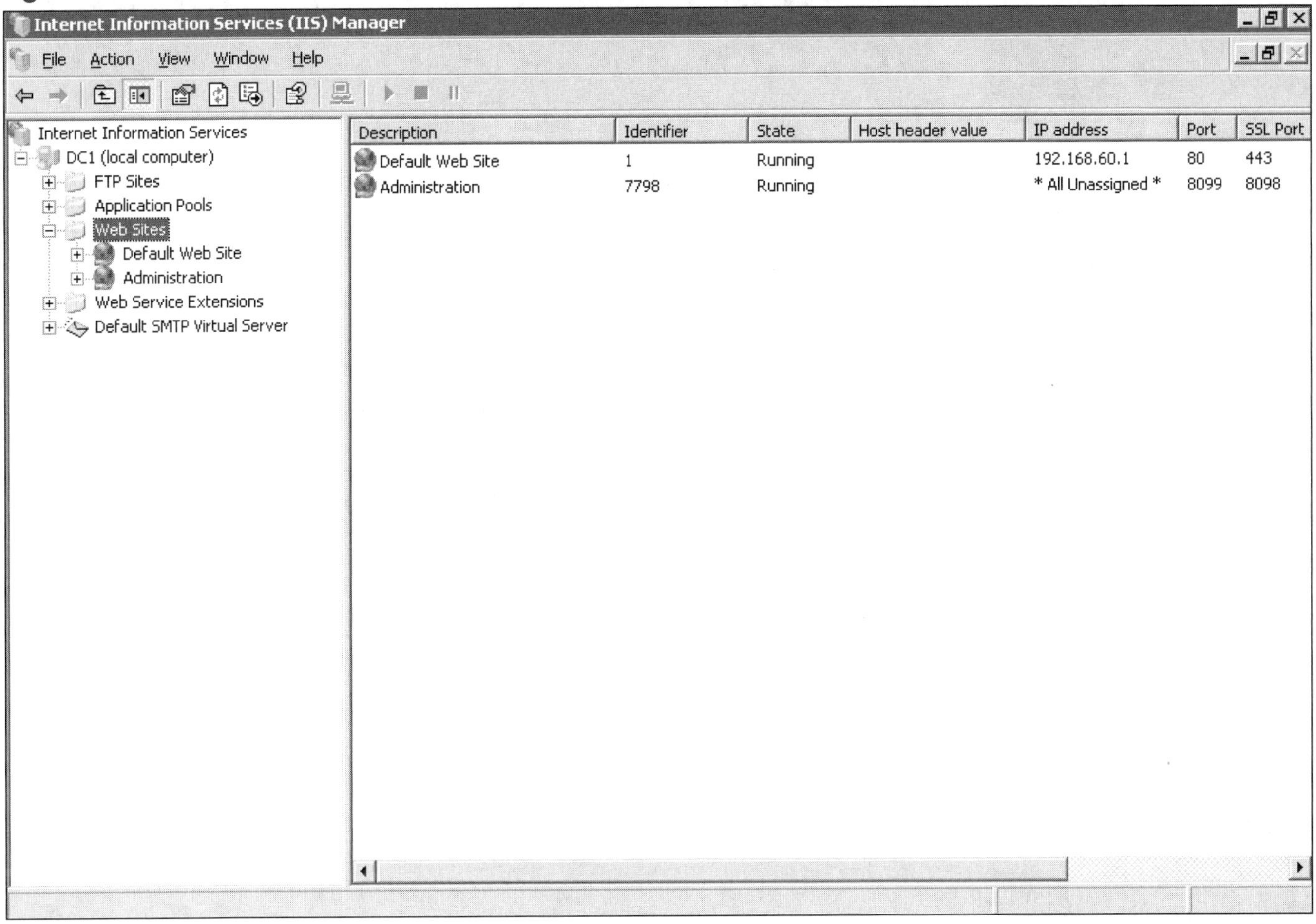

Figure 14-7 Selecting the log file format

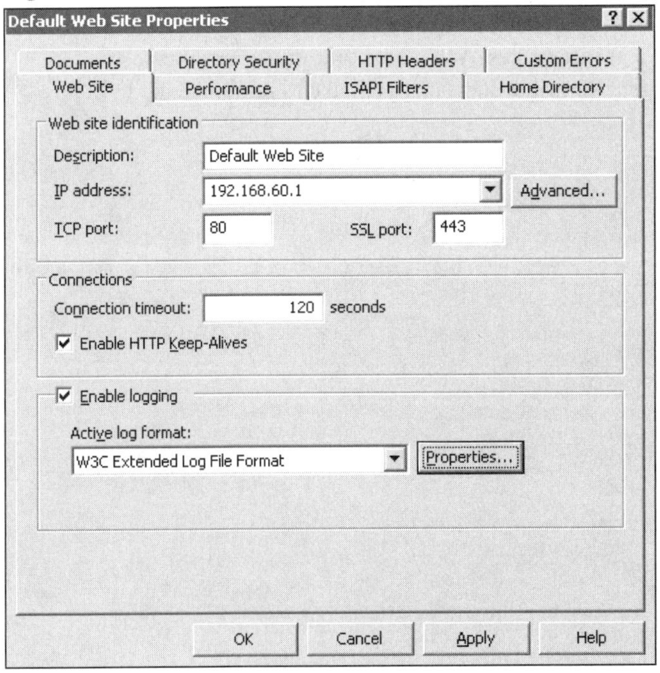

Figure 14-8 Selecting the log schedule

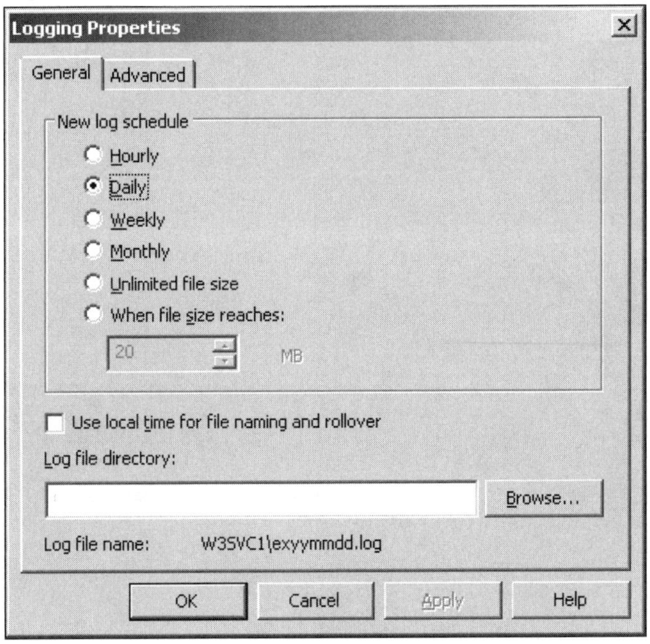

project 14.4

Designing User Authentication for a Web Site

exam objective

Design security for Internet Information Services (IIS).

Design user authentication for Internet Information Services (IIS). Design user authentication for a Web site by using IIS authentication. Design user authentication for a Web site by using certificates.

overview

You must also determine the types of authentication to support on the Web site. You can choose between using anonymous authentication, authentication using a username and password, authentication using client certificates, or authentication using .NET passports.

Authentication options are configured on the Directory Security tab of a Web Site's Properties dialog box **(Figure 14-9)** or virtual directory. You must determine which methods are supported, the security vulnerabilities presented by each, and any special configuration requirements.

learning objective

After completing this project, you will know how to design an authentication strategy for a Web site.

specific requirements

None

estimated completion time

15 minutes

project steps

1. Prepare a PowerPoint or other form of presentation that identifies each authentication method. Make sure to note the following:
   - Potential vulnerabilities
   - Server requirements
   - Client requirements
2. If you select authentication using client certifications, will you use an internal CA or an external CA to issue the client certificates? What about the server certificate?
3. If you select Basic Authentication, what steps can you take to minimize the risk?

Figure 14-9 The Directory Security tab

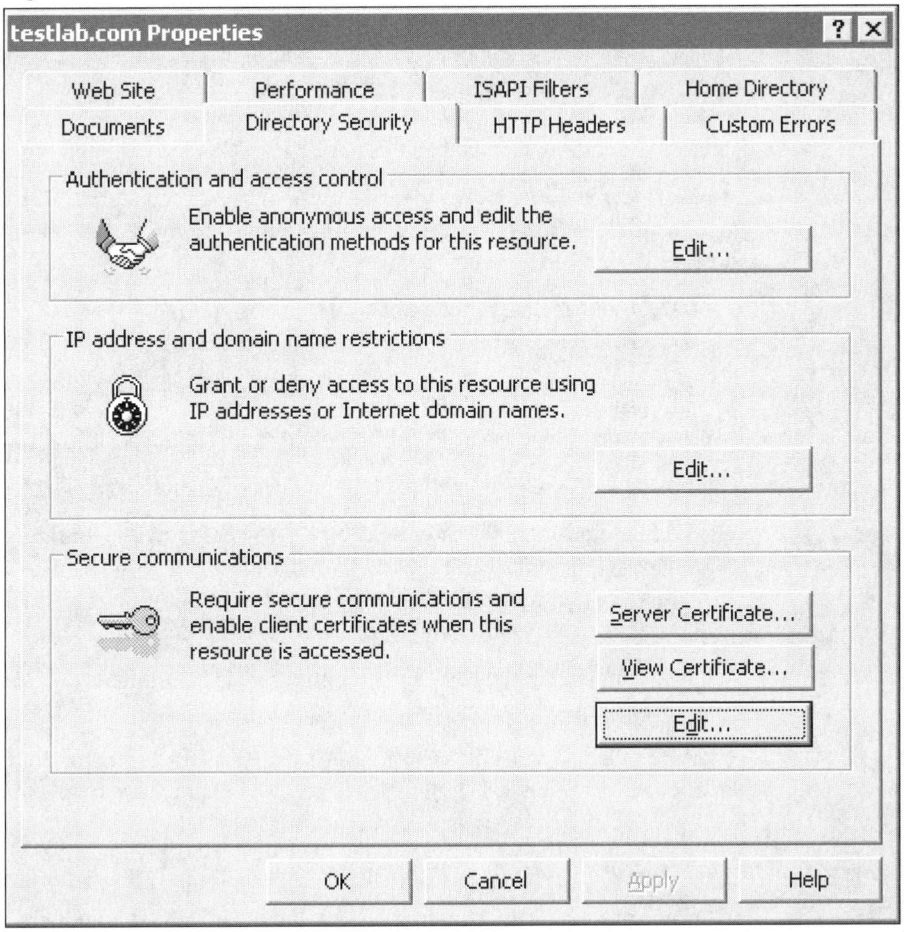

LESSON 15 Designing Security for Wireless Networks

Wireless network security is quickly becoming an inevitable part of any network security design. Even if not actively implemented as part of your network design, the fact that nearly any modern portable computer now comes with wireless networking installed and enabled means that the potential impact must be considered.

A security plan must consider wireless network concerns. The starting point is an understanding of the technologies and potential security shortcomings involved. There are three basic standards currently in use:

- **802.11b (WiFi)**: Operates at 2.4 GHz and supports 11 Mbps.
- **802.11a**: Less commonly used standard operating at 5.725-5.875 GHz and supporting 54 Mbps.
- **802.11g**: Current de facto standard operating at 2.4 GHz and supporting 54 Mbps, also supporting downward compatibility with 802.11b devices.

Wireless networks support two potential modes of operation:

- **Ad hoc mode**: This is essentially a peer-to-peer network configuration in which wireless devices communicate directly with each other.
- **Infrastructure mode**: Typically used for integrating wired and wireless networks, connections are made through wireless access points (WAPs).

Wireless-enabled computers can be configured to be limited to ad hoc only, infrastructure only, or can support both modes.

A WAP is identified by its Service Set Identifier (SSID), sometimes called the Extended Service Set Identifier (ESSID), which is set to a default value by the manufacturer. A wireless device connects to a WAP by selecting it by its SSID.

There are two supported authentication methods:

- **Open system authentication**: This is the default and does not provide any authentication but can use the wireless client Media Access Control (MAC) address for identification. By default, any client is authenticated and allowed to connect to the network.
- **Wired Equivalent Privacy (WEP)**: This is a shared key authentication method (64-bit and 128-bit keys supported) using a shared value for authentication and data encryption. The value is entered manually or generated from a supplied pass phrase value.

These methods control client authentication for enabling the client to join the wireless network. User account authentication is managed separately, the same as for traditional wired clients. However, a hacker gaining access to the wireless network could possibly capture network traffic without having to log on to network resources.

Open system authentication can be bypassed if a hacker captures a valid client's MAC address or introduces rogue (unauthorized) WAPs into the network. WEP is considered a marginally secure method at best and can be easily broken by a determined hacker.

Other problems inherent in the 802.11 standard include:

- No security identification of clients or other WAPs
- Manual key management (no completely automated management)
- Potentially weak WEP keys
- No extended authentication support, such as smart cards or certificates
- No integrated data integrity support

The 802.1x standard was developed to help address 802.11 security issues, adding client authentication support through Extensible Authentication Protocol (EAP) for passwords and digital certificates. It is a flexible standard designed to support new authentication methods as they are developed.

Access through 802.1x is based on:

- **Supplicants:** Client attempting to access the network and providing authentication credentials.
- **Authenticator:** WAP enforcing authentication and allowing access to services and protocols requested by the supplicant.
- **Authentication server:** Device authenticating the client credentials, a role performed by the WAP or a separate server dedicated to that purpose (such as a RADIUS server).

The 802.1x specification defines standards for both authenticating the client and for authorizing the protocols the client is allowed to use on the network, such as Hypertext Transfer Protocol (HTTP), Dynamic Host Configuration Protocol (DHCP), Post Office Protocol (POP)3, Simple Mail Transfer Protocol (SMTP), and so forth). It helps to close some of the holes inherent in the 802.11 standard.

Scenario

Increased use of wireless-enabled devices on the network means that wireless security must be integrated into the network design. The plan should allow mobile users and telecommuters to connect to the wired office network via wireless connections using one or more WAPs. It is important to secure network access and prevent unauthorized connections to the network.

Lesson 15 Designing Security for Wireless Networks

Project	*Exam 70-298 Objective*
15.1 Designing Public and Private Wireless LANs	**Design security for wireless networks**. Design public and private wireless LANs.
15.2 Using 802.1x Authentication for Wireless Networks	**Design security for wireless networks**. Design 802.1x authentication for wireless networks.

General Requirements

There are no special requirements for this lesson. However, you may find it helpful to refer to Lesson 15 in your Prentice Hall Certification Series Exam 70-298 textbook for additional information about the topics covered by the projects in this lesson.

project 15.1

Designing Public and Private Wireless LANs

exam objective

Design security for wireless networks. Design public and private wireless LANs.

overview

Wireless device support has become a critical, top-priority issue. The wireless security plan will be implemented throughout the United States division as soon as it is developed. Very little time has been allocated for testing before implementation. You must determine:

- Technologies currently in use **(Table 15-1)**
- Appropriate configuration mode **(Figure 15-1)**
- Appropriate authentication type

You suspect that some mobile computer users are already sharing files with each other through an unauthorized rogue "shadow" network. In other words, you suspect that mobile users are operating as a peer-to-peer ad hoc mode network running in parallel to the corporate network. You have no administrative or security control over this shadow network.

learning objective

After completing this project, you will understand guidelines for configuring wireless LANs.

specific requirements

None

estimated completion time

15 minutes

project steps

1. What is the appropriate mode type for integrating the wireless computers with the existing wired LAN?
2. How should mode support be configured for the wireless computers?
3. There is a concern about possible data entry errors when entering shared keys. Refer to **Figure 15-2** and identify the most appropriate method for entering WEP key information to avoid this problem.
4. Sketch a simple representation of the wired/wireless network design. Include a description of how the network can be expanded to support additional wireless users.

Figure 15-1 IEEE 802.11 wireless standards

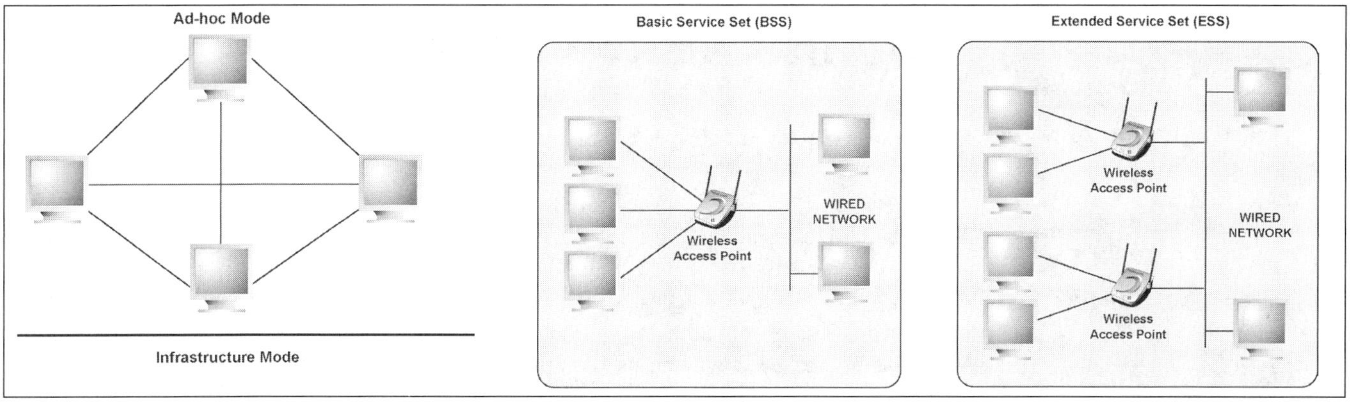

Table 15-1 IEEE 802.11 wireless standards

Standard	Frequency Range	Maximum Data (MDTR) Transmission Rate	Comments
802.11b Known as "Wi-Fi"	2.4 GHz	11 Mbps	Subject to interference with common electronic devices, such as cordless phones, microwaves, baby monitors, wireless video cameras, and Bluetooth devices.
802.11a	5.725–5.875 GHz	54 Mbps	Not as subject to common electronic devices as 802.11b. Compatibility issues with 802.11b devices. Provides higher data rate and cleaner signal than 802.11b because they are not on the same frequency as other devices (baby monitors, cordless phones, etc.)
802.11g	2.4 GHz	54 Mbps	Said to be 100% compatible with 802.11b devices. A hybrid of 802.11a and 802.11b standards.

Figure 15-2 Infrastructure and ad hoc modes

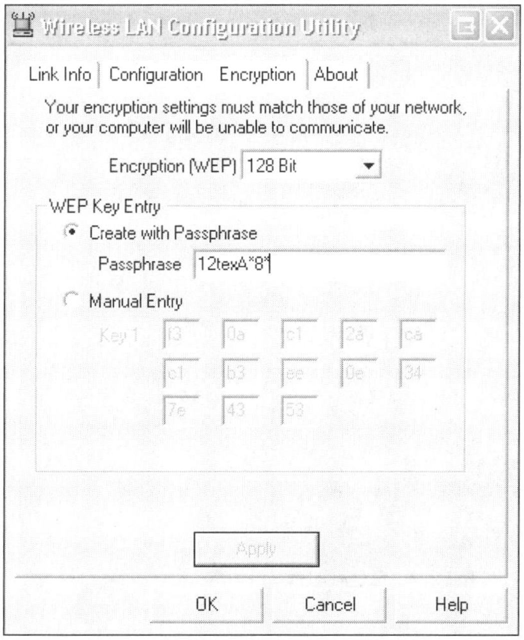

project 15.2

Using 802.1x Authentication for Wireless Networks

exam objective

Design security for wireless LANs. Design 802.1x authentication for wireless networks.

overview

You are asked to prepare a suggested networking design for small remote offices opened in the future. The plan is to configure small offices as nearly wireless-only (minimize wired connections) and provide access to the corporate enterprise network through a shared VPN connection. The proposed network model is shown in **Figure 15-3**. A computer running Windows Server 2003 will be used as the router and VPN end-point in the remote office. The server running Windows Server 2003 will use a wired connection to the local network.

You must determine the most appropriate authentication type for the design **(Table 15-2)**. The design must be as secure as possible, pass authentication information over a secure channel, and require mutual authentication.

learning objective

After completing this project, you will understand guidelines for security wireless LANs using 802.1x.

specific requirements

None, but you will need to refer to concepts presented in earlier lessons.

estimated completion time

10 minutes

project steps

1. What is the most appropriate EAP authentication type? Justify your choice by describing the shortcomings in other authentication types.
2. Justify placement of the RADIUS servers used for authentication in the Chicago office.
3. Would certificates needed in the design be provided an internal certificate authority or a public certificate authority? Why?

Table 15-2 EAP authentication types

Type	Comments
Extensible Authentication Protocol-Message Digest 5 (EAP-MD5)	Not a good option for wireless LANs because it does not support mutual authentication or automatic distribution of updates of WEP keys.
Extensible Authentication Protocol-Transport Layer Security (EAP-TLS)	Provides certificate-based authentication and mutual authentication capabilities through an encrypted tunnel. It can be used to derive per-user dynamic WEP keys and also supports per-session keys. Requires both a client and server-side certificate.
Lightweight Extensible Authentication Protocol (LEAP)	Used by CISCO WLANS. It supports dynamic WEP keys and mutual authentication.
Protected Extensible Authentication Protocol (PEAP)	Supports passing legacy password-based protocols over 802.11 wireless networks. It uses tunneling between the client and the authentication server. Requires a service side certificate but not a certificate on the client.

Figure 15-3 Wireless LAN using RADIUS

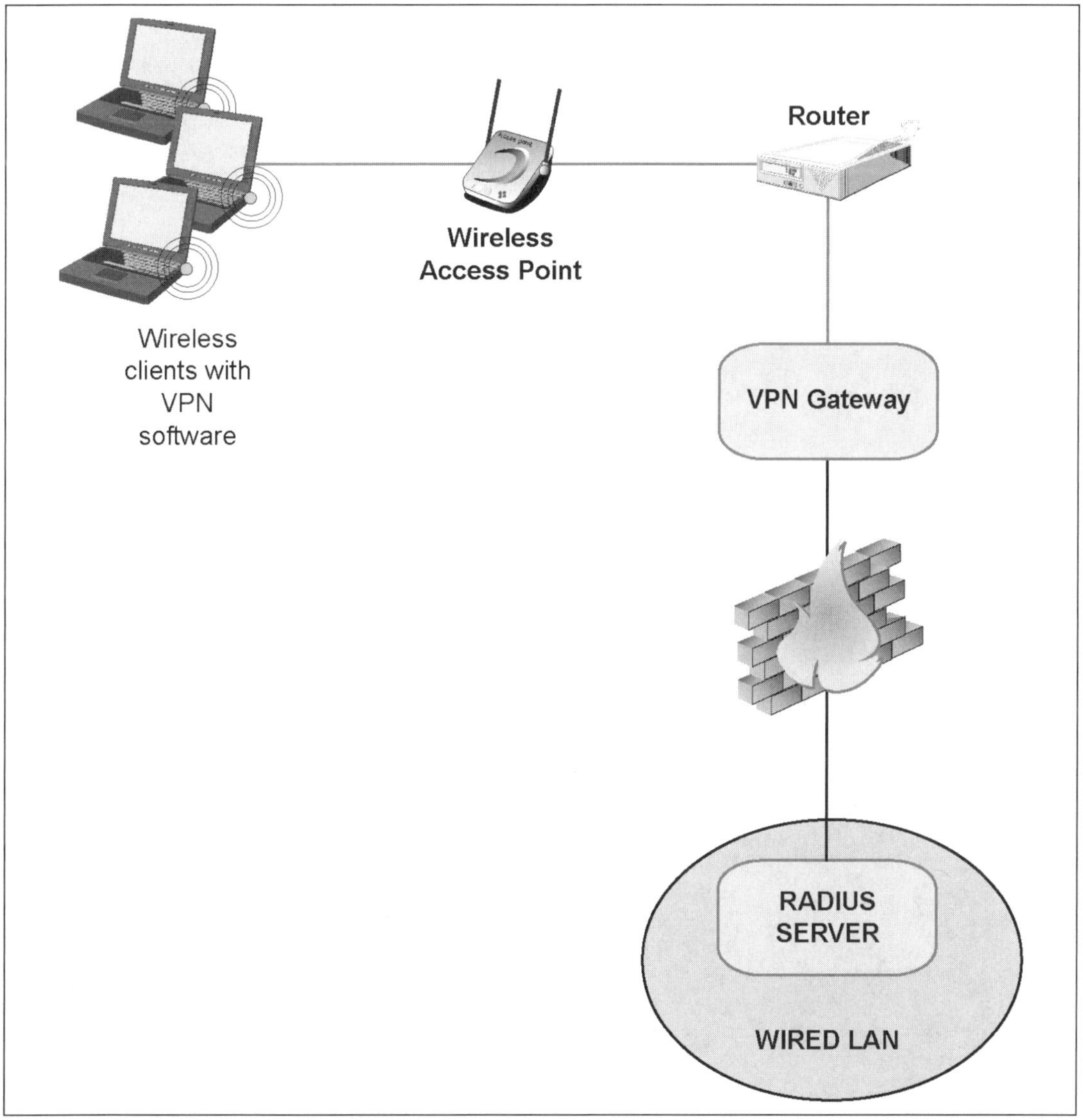

15.8 Notes

Glossary

1-to-1 mapping User submits a certificate to a Web server, which compares the copy it holds with the certificate received from the browser. If they match, the user is authenticated. If the user receives a new certificate at some later time, the mapping must be recreated once again because the certificates no longer match. 1-to-1 mappings are an excellent way to control and monitor who can access an SSL-enabled Web site.

Access control entry (ACE) Identifies the security principles and their associated rights on a resource.

Access control list (ACL) Contains security identifiers (SIDs) as well as access rights and permissions granted to the security principal.

Access token Contains the user's security identifier (SID), SIDs for any groups of which the user is a member, and the user's privileges.

Account policies Define security on domain and local accounts. Account policies contain three categories of configuration: Password Policy, Account Lockout Policy, and Kerberos Policy.

Active Directory Client Extensions Extensions for the Windows 95, Windows 98, and Windows NT 4.0 operating systems that allow those client platforms to take advantage of features provided by the Windows 2000 Active Directory service. Some of these features include NT Lan Manager version 2 authentication support and access to Windows distributed file system (Dfs) fault tolerant and fail-over file shares.

Active Server Pages (ASP) Provides the ability to integrate scripting that runs on an IIS server inside the HTML code in the Web page.

ASP.NET Enables programmers to develop Web applications using less code, and supports multiple programming languages.

Ad hoc mode A topology in which the wireless local area network is created by the wireless devices themselves.

Administrative Templates Text files that specify Registry settings that adjust various aspects of the computer's configuration or the user's desktop environment.

Advanced digest authentication Uses the same hashing process as digest authentication, but does not require that the user's password be stored using reversible encryption. The MD5 hashed password stored in Active Directory can be checked against the hashed password sent by IIS 6. Also does not require subauthentication. Can be used if both the domain controller and the IIS server are running Windows Server 2003 and the domain functional level is set to Windows Server 2003.

Advanced Encryption Standard (AES) An algorithm adopted by the U.S. government for protection of classified data in June 2003, which supports key sizes of 128,192, and 256 bits.

AES See Advanced Encryption Standard.

AH See Authentication Header.

ALE See Annual loss expectancy.

Algorithm See Cipher.

Annual loss expectancy (ALE) The total amount of money a company will lose in one year if a risk is not addressed.

Annual rate of occurrence (ARO) The number of times you expect a risk to occur in one year.

Anonymous authentication Allows users to connect to a Web site without entering any credentials. IIS uses the IUSR_Computername account to determine their access to resources.

Answering router The router in a demand-dial routing implementation that listens for connection requests from a calling router. Performs the role of the VPN server.

ARO See Annual rate of occurrence.

ASP See Active Server Pages.

ASR See Automated System Recovery.

Asymmetric key cryptography Uses a key pair (public/private) for encryption and decryption purposes.

Audit policy Identifies the types of security-related events to be recorded on computers in a network.

Auditing Enables an administrator to detect intrusions, provide accountability for user actions, and create audit trails to be used as evidence in prosecutions, as well as reconstruct how attacks occurred by recording events in various logs.

Authenticating switch A switch that prevents physical layer access by functioning as a RADIUS client. The switch performs authentication by using IAS as the authentication provider.

Authentication The process of validating the credentials of a person, computer process, or device.

Authentication Header (AH) Protocol used with IPSec that provides authentication and data integrity by digitally signing packet. Does not provide data encryption or confidentiality. It only ensures that the correct, unmodified data is sent to the correct recipient.

Authentication server This entity is responsible for checking the credentials received from the authenticator. The results (authorized/not authorized) are returned to the authenticator.

Authentication Service (AS) Component of the Key Distribution Center (KDC) in Kerberos. It is responsible for validating user credentials with Active Directory.

Authenticator A port on a wireless device that enforces authentication before it allows access to services that use the port.

Authorization The process of granting a person, computer process, or device access to certain information, functionality, or services.

Automated System Recovery (ASR) Windows 2003 tool that allows you to back up and restore the computer to its original state prior to a failure.

Automatic Updates service The client-side component of Software Update Services (SUS).

Autonomy The ability of network administrators to independently manage all or part of the directory services and all or part of the data stored in directories or member servers joined to the directory.

Available network Wireless network that is in range of the wireless network adapter. Also referred to as a known network.

Back door A hole deliberately left in the security of a system.

Base CRL Contains a complete listing of all revoked certificates and are published weekly by default.

Baseline template A template that is used to standardize security settings across all Windows Server 2003 computers in the enterprise. Its primary goal is to restrict as many settings as possible while still allowing the server to function.

Basic authentication Allows users to connect to a Web site after entering a valid user name and password.

Basic Service Set (BSS) A single wireless access point that supports one or more wireless clients.

Beacon frames Special wireless frames, transmitted several times a second and includes the device's SSID.

Bidirectional trust Two trust relationships, one in each direction.

Biometrics The science of using biological properties to identify individuals (finger prints, retinal scans, voice recognition).

Bluetooth An alternative to IEEE 802.11 wireless standards. Designed for personal digital assistants (PDAs), cellular phones, and pagers. Transmits in 2.45 GHz range, maximum range of 10 meters, and a data transmission rate of 1-2 Mbps.

Brute force attack Attempts to crack a password by using every possible password until the correct one is found.

Buffer overruns An attack in which a hacker exploits an unchecked buffer in a program and then overwrites the program's code with his or her own.

C# Pronounced *c-sharp*. This is a compiled, object oriented programming language that is used for Web applications that use the Microsoft.NET framework. It is derived from the C programming language and is used for server-side processing of ASP.NET applications. C# Web applications are usually compiled as Dynamic link library (DLL) files that are stored on the Web server.

CA See Certification Authority.

Cache poisoning The process of injecting false information into a DNS server's cache.

Cacls.exe A utility that enables you to both display and modify discretionary access control lists (DACLs) for one or more files at the same time.

Calling router Performs the role of the VPN client in a demand-dial routing implementation. The calling router waits to be authenticated and authorized by the answering router before it can forward data packets.

Canonical order The preferred order of access control entries (ACEs) in a discretionary access control list (DACL).

CAPolicy.inf A configuration file used to implement constraints when qualified subordination is used to provide trusts between public key infrastructures (PKIs).

CDFS Acronym for read-only file system for CD-ROMs.

CDP See Content distribution point.

CDP server Server that can be used to store security updates.

Centralized binary logging When this type of logging is used, all sites on the Web server write their data to a single centralized binary log file. If any site is configured with a different logging format, it is disabled on the server. This approach is more efficient than having each Web site server write its own log file in ASCII text format and consumes much less CPU and memory resources because the computer writes in binary, its native language.

Certificate See Digital certificate.

Certificate chaining A sequence of certificates, where the subsequent certificate signs each certificate in the chain. Certificate chaining is used to validate certificates.

Certificate enrollment Process by which security principals make certificate requests. Windows Server 2003 supports both manual and automatic certificate enrollment methods.

Certificate policy A document that focuses on digital certificates and the organization's responsibilities regarding these certificates. It defines how certificates are used, the process for enrolling and issuing them, and liability issues should the Certification Authority (CA) be compromised.

Certificate practice statement This document focuses on the Certification Authority (CA), the policies implemented on the CA, procedures and processes for issuing, renewing, and revoking certificates, algorithms, and key length information for the CA.

Certificate Request Wizard (CRW) A wizard that guides you through the process of enrolling and renewing a certificate with an enterprise Certification Authority.

Certificate Revocation List (CRL) A list of revoked certificates.

Certificate Revocation List Distribution Point (CDP) A location from which the Certificate Revocation List can be downloaded.

Certificate Services A service that provides the ability to issue, use, and manage digital certificates.

Certificate templates Certificates that have a pre-specified format. The content of certificate templates is based on their intended usage.

Certification Authority (CA) Organizations that issue and manage digital certificates. A CA can also refer to the computer and its associated software used to manage certificates.

Certification hierarchy An organized collection of Certification Authorities (CAs).

Chain of custody Documenting and labeling evidence with the names of those who handle it.

Cipher The set of instructions that explains how the data will actually be encrypted and decrypted. Also referred to as an algorithm.

Cipher.exe A command line utility that displays or alters the encryption on folders and files on NTFS partitions.

Ciphertext Plaintext that has been encrypted using an encryption algorithm.

Cluster A group of independent systems, physically connected with cabling and logically connected through cluster software, that work together to run applications.

Common Gateway Interface (CGI) script/executable A program that is executed in real-time to provide dynamic output in response to user input.

Compulsory tunnel A tunnel created to send data between two virtual private network routers in a site-to-site demand-dial configuration. It is considered compulsory because no other routes are used to transport the data.

Computer Security Incident Response Team (CSIRT) A group of people with the needed skills to address security incidents.

Configuration partition/naming context Contains information about which domains exist in the forest, which domain controllers are located in those domains as well as the available services. This partition is replicated to all domain controllers in the entire forest.

Console redirection Allows your computer to send text information to the out-of-band.

Content distribution point (CDP) In situations where areas of your network do not have access to the Internet, you must provide a way to deliver security updates. This can be accomplished by creating a CDP on a server to store the security updates.

Content management server A server running Internet Information Services (IIS) 5.0 or later that acts as a storage point for security updates that are copied from a running Software Update Services (SUS) server.

CRL See Certificate Revocation List.

Cross-certification trust The process where a public key infrastructure (PKI) establishes a trust relationship with another PKI. This allows certificates presented by security principals from one PKI to be trusted in the other PKI. Also referred to as qualified subordination.

CRW See Certificate Request Wizard.

Cryptography The art of keeping messages secret.

CSIRT See Computer Security Incident Response Team.

DACL See Discretionary access control list.

Data Decryption Field (DDF) Contains the File Encryption Key (FEK) that is encrypted using the user's public key.

Data Encryption Standard (DES) An algorithm developed by International Business Machines (IBM) and adopted as a national standard in 1977. Uses a 64-bit key for encryption and decryption.

Data Recovery Agent (DRA) A user authorized to decrypt data that was encrypted by another user.

Data Recovery Field (DRF) Contains the File Encryption Key (FEK), which is encrypted with each recovery agent certificates' public key.

Dcpromo.exe The command used to start the Active Directory Installation Wizard.

DCW See Delegation of Control Wizard.

DDF See Data Decryption Field.

DDoS See Distributed Denial of Service.

Decryption The process of converting ciphertext back into plaintext.

Delegation of Control Wizard (DCW) Facilitates delegating control of different parts of Active Directory to other administrators.

Delta CRL Contains a list of certificates that have been revoked since the last base or delta CRL was published.

Demand-dial connection An on-demand connection created between two networks.

Demilitarized zone (DMZ) A network that is not part of a private network but, unlike the public Internet, is under the control of the organization that owns the network.

Denial of Service (DoS) attack This type of threat, common on Web servers, keeps legitimate users from accessing the services. A DoS attack is an element of the STRIDE acronym.

DES See Data Encryption Standard.

DHCP Relay Agent protocol A computer that broadcasts IP configuration between Dynamic Host Configuration Protocol (DHCP)-enabled clients and DHCP servers when they are on different network segments.

Dictionary file Database of common passwords derived from shared experiences of password crackers.

Diffie-Hellman (DH) key exchange protocol A protocol that demonstrates how keys can be exchanged securely over an insecure medium. The protocol is used for key distribution not for digital signatures or encryption purposes. Created by Whitfield Diffie and Martin Hellman in 1976. Also referred to as the Diffie-Hellman algorithm.

Digest authentication Improves upon basic authentication by not sending the user credentials over the network but instead sends them in the form of a Message Digest (MD) 5 hash. Requires user's password to be stored with reversible encryption.

Digital certificate Used in public key cryptography to bind the public key to the party that holds the corresponding private key. Used for encryption, nonrepudiation and authentication. Also referred to as a certificate.

Directive on Data Protection A policy established in Europe that states that "member states may transfer personal data to third countries only after the third country in question ensures adequate levels of data protection."

Disaster recovery plan A plan that can be used to recover a company from disasters.

Discretionary access control list (DACL) One or more access control entries (ACEs) that specify access rights granted to particular users or groups, each of which is identified by a security identifier (SID).

Distributed Denial of Service (DDoS) The use of multiple remote systems to send traffic to a single location with the goal of flooding the computer or network with traffic.

Distributed file system (Dfs) Distributes and integrates file shares located on multiple computers into a single logical namespace. It is required for Active Directory's SYSVOL share. SYSVOL relies on the proper operation of Dfs.

DMZ See Demilitarized zone.

DNS See Domain Name System.

DNS round-robin A load-balancing mechanism that allows requests to be distributed to multiple servers.

Domain A collection of computers, users, and groups that share a common directory database, security policies, and security relationships with other domains.

Domain Name System (DNS) The main name resolution service for Windows Server 2003 and Windows 2000.

Domain partition/naming context Contains information about objects that are specific for a domain. These include users, groups, computers, and organizational units. This partition will be replicated to all domain controllers in the same domain.

DoS See Denial of Service attack.

DRA See Data Recovery Agent.

Dynamic DNS (DDNS) Based on RFC 2136, clients can automatically update their DNS records. Domain controllers also use the capability to register their SRV records.

Dynamic link library (DLL) files A file that contains a collection of Windows functions that perform a specific task when called upon by a program.

EAP-TLS See Extensible Authentication Protocol-Transfer Layer Protocol.

EFS See Encrypting File System.

Efsinfo.exe Command-line tool that displays information about files and folders encrypted with Encrypting File System (EFS) on NTFS partitions.

Elevation of privilege This threat occurs when an attacker convinces a system that he or she should have administrative-level privileges. An attacker who is able to gain elevated privileges might be able to use those privileges to gain access to other applications running on the computer. Elevation of privilege is an element of the STRIDE acronym.

Electronic tape vaulting Replaces manual backup and tape transport with electronic transmission of backup data to remote tape drives.

Emergency Management Services (EMS) A new feature in Windows Server 2003 that provides remote administration using out-of-band connections.

Emergency Repair Disk (ERD) A disk used to repair the startup environment, verify and replace missing and damaged system files, and inspect and repair the boot sector.

EMS See Emergency Management Services.

Encapsulating Security Payload (ESP) An Internet Protocol Security (IPSec) protocol used to provide encryption. It provides data integrity and confidentiality for IPSec. See RFC 1827 for more details.

Encrypting File System (EFS) A feature introduced in Windows 2000 that enables users to encrypt and decrypt files on NTFS partitions.

Encryption The process of scrambling plaintext into a form that cannot be read by others.

End-to-end encryption Encryption of information over the entire path between two computers.

Enrollment agent An individual who requests certificates on behalf of another security principal.

Enterprise CA Publishes certificates and CRLs using information in Active Directory, such as user accounts and security group information, to approve or deny requests for certificates.

ERD See Emergency Repair Disk.

ESP See Encapsulating Security Payload.

ESS See Extended Service Set.

Explicit permission Permissions that are attached directly to an object, either when it is created or by user action.

Extended Service Set (ESS) A set of two or more wireless access points that are connected to the same wired network.

Extensible Authentication Protocol-Transport Layer Protocol (EAP-TLS) Enables mutual authentication between the client and server computers in a VPN connection.

External trust A trust relationship established between a Windows Server 2003 domain and an NT4 domain or between Windows Server 2003 domains in separate forests.

Federal Information Processing Standards (FIPS) Publicly announced standards developed by the U. S. government for use by all (non-military) government agencies and by government contractors. Example: Data Encryption Standard (FIPS 46).

File Encryption Key (FEK) Randomly generated symmetric key.

File Replication Service (FRS) Enables files to be automatically copied and maintained simultaneously on multiple servers.

File Transfer Protocol (FTP) service Utilizes the File Transfer Protocol to exchange files between computers.

Filter Tells IPSec what type of traffic to apply the filter action to. A filter is stored in the IP filter list of the policy.

Filter action Determine what should be done with traffic that matches a filter in the IPSec policy.

Firewall A device that protects resources on a private network from users of other networks.

Firmware Programming that is inserted into Programmable Read-Only Memory (PROM).

Footprinting The process of capturing network information that can be used for future attacks.

Forest A group of one or more domains that share a common schema, global catalog, and configuration. All domains in the forest have a two-way transitive trust relationship.

Forest trust A trust relationship between two Windows Server 2003 forest root domains.

FrontPage Server Extensions Server-side extensions that are a companion to FrontPage, a Microsoft program used to create and edit HTML documents. Allows direct access to Web folders on remote server for authoring and administration functions.

FRS See File Replication Service.

FTP User Isolation Prevents users from viewing or overwriting content stored in other directories.

Generic Route Encapsulation (GRE) Allows one network protocol to be transferred over the network inside another network protocol. Synonymous with Point-to-Point Tunneling Protocol (PPTP).

Global catalog server A domain controller that stores updatable directory partitions (full replica) and a read only copy of the domain partition for all other domains in the same forest (partial replica).

Global Positioning Satellite (GPS) receiver Locates four or more earth orbiting satellites, determines the distance to each, and then uses the information to determine its own location.

GPMC See Group Policy Management Console.

GPO See Group Policy Object.

Gpupdate.exe A command-line utility that enables you to force the refresh of Group Policy settings on a computer rather than wait for the default refresh period to be reached.

Gramm-Leach-Bliley Financial Modernization Act of 1999 Requires that financial and insurance institutions disclose to customers their policies for protecting the privacy of non-public personal information.

Group Policy A set of configuration settings applied by administrators to objects in Active Directory.

Group Policy Management Console (GPMC) A console that is designed to simplify the management of Group Policy by providing a single location for managing all aspects of Group Policy settings. Prior to GPMC, administrators had to use several tools to manage Group Policy. GPMC integrates those tools into a single console and also provides backup/restore capabilities, HTML reporting capabilities, and simulation and modeling possibilities. The tool is not on the Windows Server 2003 CD; you must download it from Microsoft.

Group Policy Object (GPO) A collection of Group Policy settings. The GPO can be linked to a site, domain, or organizational unit, and affect users and computers in those containers.

Hardware security module Used to protect key pairs and sign issued certificates. Provides the ability to remove the key pairs for a Certification Authority (CA) and store them in a safer place.

Hash value Provides data integrity for the message. It is a number generated from a string of text by using a formula which multiples two large prime numbers. Also referred to as a message digest.

Hashing The process of running some portion of a message through a one-way hashing algorithm that produces output known as a hash value or message digest. The hashing algorithm takes a variable-length text string as input and produces a fixed-length binary value as output. The hashing function is called one-way because it is theoretically impossible to take the output (hashing value) and determine the input needed to create the message digest. Message digests verify the integrity of messages to ensure that they have not been modified while in transit. Examples of popular hashing algorithms include Message Digest 5 (MD5) and Secure Hash Algorithm 1 (SHA-1).

Hashing function Mathematical formula that converts a message into a fixed-length string of digits, referred to as a hash value or message digest.

Headless server A server that can be managed without a local display or input devices.

Health Insurance Portability and Accountability Act (HIPAA) Legislation designed to improve the security and privacy of shared medical information.

Hot fix A single file or multiple files that can be applied to an operating system to correct a specific problem. Released in between service packs.

HTTP SSL service Uses Secure Sockets Layer (SSL) to encrypt and decrypt requests for Web pages as well as the pages actually sent back to the user.

IAS See Internet Authentication Service.

IBSS See Independent Basic Service Set.

ICV See Integrity check value.

IDS See Intrusion detection system.

IEAK See Internet Explorer Administration Kit.

IEEE See Institute of Electrical and Electronic Engineers.

IEEE 802.1x Introduced to address issues with authentication and optionally, key management. It uses EAP to transport authentication traffic between the wireless client and an authentication server.

IEEE 802.11b Created in July 1999 for the home user market. Is currently the most widespread standard in use, but uses the unregulated 2.4 GHz frequency range shared by several common electrical devices, such as 2.5 GHz cordless phones, copiers, and microwaves.

IEEE 802.11a Created at the same time as 802.11b but marketed to the business sector, IEEE 802.11a supports up to 54 Mbps and uses the 5 GHz frequency range. Because 802.11a and 802.11b use different frequencies, they are incompatible with each other.

IEEE 802.11g A hybrid version of 802.11a and 802.11b. Was introduced in late 2002 and became a standard in 2003. It supports the higher data throughput rate of 54 Mbps (802.11a) and uses the 2.4 GHz frequency (801.11b) for better range. Higher frequencies do not pass through walls and other obstacles as well as lower frequencies. 802.11g is also backward compatible with 802.11b. This means that you can use an 802.11g wireless access point (WAP) with 802.11b wireless network adapters and vice versa. 802.11b wireless adapters cannot have their firmware upgraded to 802.11g capabilities but instead must be replaced.

IEEE 802.11i An Institute of Electrical and Electronics Engineers (IEEE) standard for security in a wireless local area network. 802.11i will replace the Wi-Fi Protected Access (WPA version 1) encryption protocol, which is considered very insecure, with Advanced Encryption Standard (AES), a much more computing-intensive algorithm. Also known as WPA version 2.

Identity Integration Server 2003 A centralized server service that stores and integrates identity information for organizations with multiple directories. It provides a unified view of all known identity information about users, applications, and network resources.

IIS See Internet Information Services.

IIS Admin service Required for an IIS server to run Web, File Transfer Protocol (FTP), Network News Transfer Protocol (NNTP), or Simple Mail Transfer Protocol (SMTP) services or configure IIS. It provides a way for services to access and manage the IIS metabase.

IIS 5.0 Lockdown Tool A wizard-based tool that provides the ability to turn off unnecessary features which reduces the attack surface on IIS.

IIS Manager utility A graphical interface for configuring Internet Information Services.

IIS metabase A plain-text, XML data store that contains IIS configuration information.

IKE See Internet Key Exchange.

In-band connections Standard connections an administrator would use to connect to another computer over the network or via its local console.

Incident response plan A plan that provides procedures responding to security incidents.

Incident response procedure Includes a purpose statement that defines the purpose of the procedure, a scope statement that defines the area the procedure covers, and a definition of incident statement that describes what represents an incident. Also defines areas of responsibilities, and describes how to classify incidents and the appropriate response measures, the appropriate procedure for, and handling evidence, and the details that need to be documented regarding the incident.

Incremental template A template used to modify settings implemented in the baseline template so that a server can perform its specified role. In most cases, this means enabling services that have been disabled via the baseline template.

Independent Basic Service Set (IBSS) An ad hoc wireless network in which wireless clients create a local area network (LAN) among themselves without the use of a wireless access point (WAP).

Information disclosure This threat results when information is made available to individuals who are not authorized to view it. Information disclosure is an element of the STRIDE acronym.

Infrastructure mode Extends the wired network to wireless devices by implementing a wireless access point.

Inheritance Process by which any new files and subfolders created in a folder inherit permissions that have been set on a parent folder.

Inherited permission Permission propagated to an object from a parent object.

Initialization vector (IV) A number that, in addition to the encryption key, provides randomness to the encryption process.

Institute of Electrical and Electronic Engineers (IEEE) An international organization that develops standards for hundreds of electronic and electrical technologies.

Integrated Windows authentication Uses Kerberos for authentication. This authentication method is limited to Internet Explorer browsers only and does not work over HTTP proxy connections.

Integrity check value (ICV) A checksum value that is used to detect packet modification.

Intermediary CA See Subordinate CA.

Internet Authentication Service (IAS) Microsoft's implementation of a Remote Authentication Dial-In User Service (RADIUS) server and proxy and is described in Request for Comments (RFC) 2865.

Internet Authentication Service snap-in Snap-in used to manage the Internet Authentication Service (IAS).

Internet Data Connector (IDC) A tool that sends queries to a database, formats the data retuned into HTML, and then sends the page to the user's browser.

Internet Explorer Administration Kit (IEAK) A toolkit available from Microsoft that includes the Internet Explorer Customization Wizard and the IEAK Profile Manager. These components allow you to customize, deploy and manage Internet Explorer.

Internet Information Services (IIS) Microsoft's Web server software.

Internet Key Exchange (IKE) A combination of two protocols: the Internet Security Association and Key Management Protocol (ISAKMP) and the Oakley Key Determination protocol. Used during security association negotiations in IPSec negotiation policies.

Internet Protocol Security (IPSec) A suite of network layer protocols that extends the Internet Protocol (IP) by providing mechanisms for authentication, confidentiality, and integrity in IP-based communications.

Internet Storm Center A subsidiary of the SANS Institute. It gathers more than 3,000,000 intrusion detection logs every day and uses them to monitor Internet traffic, isolate the sites that are used for attacks, and provides authoritative data on the types of attacks being mounted against computers in industries and regions worldwide.

Interoperability The ability of software and hardware on different computers from different vendors to share information.

Intrusion detection system (IDS) Monitors packets as they travel through the network looking for suspicious patterns that might indicate an attack is in progress.

Intrusion prevention system (IPS) Monitors packets as they travel through the network looking for suspicious patterns that might indicate an attack is in progress. This type of system can also respond to an actual attack by programming the firewall to block traffic or terminating the connection.

IP spoofing A technique used by attackers to gain unauthorized access to computes. The intruder sends messages to a computer with an IP address that indicates the message is coming from a trusted host.

IPSec See Internet Protocol Security.

IPSec Network Address Translation Traversal (IPSec NATT) Provides a way for two computers to detect that a NAT device is present between them and begin encapsulating IPSec packets inside of UDP packets over port 4500.

IPSec policy Used to implement IPSec. It consists of rules, filters, and filter actions.

IPSec Security Association (SA) A combination of a policy and keys that defines the common security services, mechanisms, and keys used to protect the communication from end to end.

IPSec transport mode An IPSec configuration parameter that encrypts traffic between a client and server.

IPSec tunnel mode An IPSec configuration parameter that encrypts traffic between two endpoints.

Isolation The ability of network administrators to prevent other administrators from controlling or interfering with delivery of directory services and/or data stored in directories or members servers joined to the directory.

Issuing CA Provides certificates to users, computes, and services (security principals).

IV See Initialization vector.

KDC See Key Distribution Center.

Kerberos An authentication protocol developed by the Massachusetts Institute of Technology. Microsoft introduced it in its release of Windows 2000.

Kerberos realm A realm consists of applications and services that use the Kerberos authentication protocols and a Key Distribution Center (KDC). Similar to a domain, users belong to a specific Kerberos realm.

Kernel The core of the Windows operating system. It provides basic services for all other parts of the operating system.

Key A combination of alpha and/or numeric characters that can be used by an algorithm to customize the transformation of plaintext into ciphertext, and vice versa.

Key Distribution Center (KDC) The network service installed when you set up a domain controller. Provides ticket granting tickets and service tickets.

Key length Represents the number of possible combinations for the key. In modern cryptography, binary keys are used and specified in bits. The length of the key itself contributes to the vulnerability of a cipher to exhaustive search attacks.

Known network See Available network.

L2TP/IPSec See Layer Two Tunneling Protocol over IP Security.

LAN Manager An authentication protocol used by legacy version of Microsoft products. Windows 3.1, Windows for Workgroups 3.11, Windows 9x and Windows Millennium Edition.

Layer Two Tunneling Protocol over IP Security (L2TP/IPSec) A tunneling protocol used in VPNs. It is based on PPTP and L2F. It uses DES and 3DES to provide stronger encryption than does PPTP.

LCP See Link Control Protocol.

Leased lines A telecommunications service provided to companies by telephone companies and long distance carriers. It provides a permanent direct connection between two local area networks. Leased lines are available in 56 Kbps, T1, T3, and higher speeds.

Legacy system A system including hardware and software applications no longer considered state-of-the-art but are still used by the company to perform business-critical functions.

Lightweight Directory Access Protocol (LDAP) A protocol used to query directory services for information.

Link Control Protocol (LCP) Used in combination with Point-to-Point Protocol (PPP) to establish, tear down, and test a data link.

Link encryption Encryption of packets between two tunnel endpoints only.

Local Security Authority (LSA) Responsible for validating users for both local and remote logons. It queries the database for user and group SIDs and binds them to the user's access token.

LSA See Local Security Authority.

Main mode In this mode, Internet Key Exchange (IKE) decides which authentication method the computers will use. After they are authenticated, the Diffie-Helman protocol generates a shared symmetric key that is used to create a secure channel between the two systems. Also known as Phase 1.

Man-in-the-middle (MIM) attack Occurs when an attacker intercepts User A's public key when being sent to User B, and instead substitutes a different public key belonging to the attacker. User A then encrypts his or her message to User B unknowingly using the attacker's public key. When the message is sent, the attacker can intercept it, decrypt the message, view its contents, and—if desired—modify its contents. The attacker can then use User A's public key (intercepted earlier) to encrypt the contents and send it on to User A. Neither User A nor User B will know what has happened unless the information modified by attacker looks suspicious or makes no sense and generates discussions between the two.

Many-to-1 mapping Accepts all certificates that meet a specific rule that you define. Allows multiple users to authenticate through a common account.

Master DNS Server The DNS server from which a slave DNS server obtains its copy of the zone file.

Media access control (MAC) address 48-bit numbers burned into network adapters by the manufacturer. Software can be used to change wireless network adapter MAC addresses.

Message Digest 5 An algorithm used to provide data integrity with Authentication Header (AH) and Encapsulating Security Protocol (ESP).

Microsoft Baseline Security Analyzer (MBSA) Tool used to scan systems and report common security configuration vulnerabilities and determine which patches are missing.

Microsoft Challenge-Handshake Authentication Protocol (MS-CHAP) An authentication protocol used with Point-to-Point Protocol (PPP). It is a challenge/response protocol that avoids sending the user's password across the connection.

Microsoft Management Console (MMC) A framework for hosting administrative tools called snap-ins.

Microsoft Operations Framework (MOF) risk model Microsoft framework for developing a structured approach to performing risk management.

Microsoft Point-to-Point Encryption (MPPE) An encryption protocol used with Point-to-Point Tunneling Protocol (PPTP). It provides link encryption and also encrypts the Point-to-Point (PPP) payload.

Mission statement Defines why a company exists and the type of business it is in.

MMC See Microsoft Management Console.

MPPE See Microsoft Point-to-Point Encryption.

MS-CHAP See Microsoft Challenge Handshake Authentication Protocol.

Multi-master replication Multi-master means there are multiple domain controllers known as masters. Each master can modify and control the same information.

Multifactor authentication Uses three factors to authenticate: Something the user is (such as fingerprints or iris scans), something the user knows (such as passwords or personal identification number [PIN]) and something the user has (such as a token or smartcard).

Mutual authentication Authentication of both ends of a communication session.

NAQC See Network Access Quarantine Control.

NAT See Network address translation.

National Institute of Standards and Technology (NIST) An agency in the technology administration of the U.S. Department of Commerce. Its mission involves working with industry to develop and apply technology, measurements, and standards. It publishes the Federal Information Processing Standards (FIPS) and oversees the Data Encryption Standard (DES).

NDS See Novell NetWare Directory Services.

.NET Passport authentication Allows users to use a single sign-in name for every .NET Passport-enabled Web site they visit. Authentication is processed by a central database at Microsoft.

NetMeeting Conferencing software that enables real-time communication and collaboration over the Internet or intranet.

Network Access Quarantine Control (NAQC) A new feature in Windows Server 2003 that enables administrators to specify configuration conditions that must be met for a remote client to connect (service packs, security patches, antivirus software, and personal firewalls).

Network address translation (NAT) Translates IP addresses in one network into those for a different network.

Network address translator An IP router that can translate IP addresses and TCP/UDP port numbers of packets as they are forwarded. See RFC 1631 for more details.

Network News Transfer Protocol (NNTP) service Uses the Network News Transfer Protocol to host newsgroups.

Network perimeter Anywhere one network connects to another.

NIST See National Institute of Standards and Technology.

Non-transitive trust A trust that does not extend to other domains.

Novell NetWare Directory Services (NDS) A database used by Novell NetWare to organize resources for an entire network of NetWare servers. Available in NetWare 4.0 and later versions.

NT LAN Manager (NTLM) A challenge/response based authentication protocol introduced with Windows NT.

NT LAN Manager Version 2 (NTLMv2) An authentication protocol that is an enhanced version of NTLM, which was introduced in Windows NT 4. The enhanced version provides improved security and is supported by NT 4 Service Pack 4 or later.

NTFS permissions Set of permissions that restricts access to files and folders.

Office Update Microsoft's Web site for obtaining updates to its Office product suites.

On-demand connection A connection type configured on tunnel endpoints. It sets up the connection, sends the data, and after a preconfigured amount of time, terminates it.

One-way initiated connection This type of connection occurs when one router is always the calling router and the other is always the answering router.

One-way trust A trust in which one domain allows another's users access to its resources.

Open system authentication Provides identification of wireless clients through media access control addresses.

Out-of-band connections Management of a server by using a special port or device, such as a terminal concentrator or service processor.

Packet filtering A feature incorporated into routers and firewalls to limit the flow of information based on predetermined communications, such as source, destination, or type of service being provided by the network.

Passphrase Generally longer than a password and includes alphanumeric characters and symbols.

Password Policies Used for domain and local user accounts to define settings for passwords, such as enforcement, password lifetimes, and complexity settings.

PEAP See Protected Extensible Authentication Protocol.

Perimeter network See Demilitarized zone.

PERL See Practical Extraction and Reporting Language.

Persistent connection Used for connections where the link is always available. If a persistent connection is used and the connection is dropped, the server attempts to re-establish the connection.

PKI See Public Key Infrastructure.

Plaintext authentication Transmits user name and password in cleartext.

Point-to-Point Tunneling Protocol (PPTP) A protocol used to encapsulate network traffic sent across a virtual private network. It works by encapsulating Point-to-Point Protocol (PPP) packets in IP packets before sending them across the tunnel. PPTP was developed by Microsoft. See RFC 2637 for more details.

PolicySettings.xls A spreadsheet listing all Administrative Templates, their contents, and the default Registry settings for Windows XP.

PPTP See Point-to-Point Tunneling Protocol.

Practical Extraction and Reporting Language (PERL) A scripting language that can be compiled into executable files. Perl is often used for CGI programming.

Preferred network A wireless network that the client has been configured to connect and authenticate to. Are listed in order of precedence.

Principle of least privilege A basic tenet of computer security that states, "Users should be given no more privilege than necessary to perform their job functions."

Private key In asymmetric key cryptography, part of a public/private key pair. The keys are mathematically related; therefore, a message encrypted by using one key can be decrypted by using the same algorithm with the other key. When confidentiality is required, the public key is used to encrypt data and the corresponding private key to decrypt it. If authentication is required, the keys are reversed. The private key is used to sign, or encrypt the message, and the public key is used to decrypt the signature.

Probe request Frame sent when a wireless device is turned on to locate other wireless clients and wireless access points.

Promiscuous mode Enables a network to read and intercept all traffic on the network to which it is connected.

Protected Extensible Authentication Protocol (PEAP) Provides a means to protect another EAP method within a secure channel.

Proxy firewalls A device that intercepts messages leaving or entering the network and repackages them by replacing the source IP address with its own.

Public key In asymmetric key cryptography, part of a public/private key pair. The keys are mathematically related; therefore, a message encrypted using one key can be decrypted using the same algorithm with the other key. When confidentiality is required, the public key is used to encrypt data and the corresponding private key to decrypt it. If authentication is required, the keys are reversed. The private key is used to sign or encrypt the message, and the public key is used to decrypt the signature

Public Key Infrastructure (PKI) A system of digital certificates and certification authorities that verify and authenticate the validity of each party involved in electronic transactions by using public key cryptography

Qualified subordination See Cross-certification trust.

Qualitative analysis A form of risk analysis that ranks risks based on their impact on business operations and walks through different scenarios that might occur. Information received using this type of analysis is based on the experience of those involved as well as their judgment or feelings.

Quantitative analysis A form of risk analysis where actual values are placed on assets based on the probability and impact of threats.

Quick Mode In this mode, the IPSec security associations are set up. During this mode, the two systems negotiate which security algorithms they will use. Also known as Phase 2.

RADIUS See Remote Authentication Dial-In User Service.

RDA See Remote Desktop for Administration.

RDC See Remote Desktop Connection.

RDP See Remote Desktop Protocol.

Remote access policy permissions Permissions set by a remote access policy.

RADIUS authentication See Remote Authentication Dial-In User Service (RADIUS) authentication.

RADIUS client See Remote Authentication Dial-In User Service (RADIUS) client.

RADIUS proxy See Remote Authentication Dial-In User Service (RADIUS) proxy

RADIUS server See Remote Authentication Dial-In User Service (RADIUS) Server.

Realm A logical network that shares a single Kerberos database; similar to a domain.

Realm trust Used between a non-Windows Kerberos V5 realm and a Windows Server 2003 realm.

Recovery policy Identifies which user accounts are designated as data recovery agents.

Recursive queries A request from a host to a DNS server asking it to look up information in its DNS zone files.

Registry A database containing configuration and control information for a system, including information about file systems and drivers. The configuration manager helps manage registry-key objects in the database.

Registry Editor Tool used to view and manage the Registry.

Registry entry Component of the Registry. Analogous to files.

Registry key Component of the Registry. Analogous to folders.

Registry subkey Component of the Registry. Analogous to subfolders.

Remote Access Account Lockout A feature in Windows Server 2003 that can be used to protect VPN servers against dictionary-based attacks.

Remote access policy Consists of conditions, permissions, and profile settings to authenticate and authorize remote user connections.

Remote access policy conditions Connection attributes that are compared against the incoming remote access attempt.

Remote access policy permissions Permissions set by a remote access policy.

Remote access policy profile Settings in a remote access policy that specify restrictions that apply to authorized connections.

Remote Administration mode A mode used in Windows 2000 Terminal Servers that enables up to two network administrators to connect and manage the server simultaneously.

Remote Assistance A Windows Server 2003 and Windows XP utility used to invite a person to chat with you, observe your screen, and, if you give permission, to remotely control your machine to fix problems.

Remote Authentication Dial-In User Service (RADIUS) A client server protocol that allows remote access servers to communicate with a central server to authenticate dial in users and authorize their access.

Remote Authentication Dial-In User Service (RADIUS) authentication When selected as the method of authentication, the RRAS server forwards authentication requests to a RADIUS server.

Remote Authentication Dial-In User Service (RADIUS) client A dial-up server, VPN server, or WAP that is responsible for accepting the initial connection from the remote access client. It passes the request to a RADIUS server.

Remote Authentication Dial-In User Service (RADIUS) server A server that provides centralized authentication, authorization and accounting services.

Remote Desktop Connection (RDC) Client-side software used to access Terminal Servers.

Remote Desktop for Administration (RDA) A tool that enables administrators to manage Windows Server 2003 computers. It is built upon the Remote Administration mode used by Windows 2000. Terminal Services does not have to be installed to use this tool.

Remote Desktop Protocol (RDP) Enables clients to both view the output from the Terminal Server and send commands to the Terminal Server.

Remote Desktop Users Users in this group are allowed remote access to server.

Remote Procedure Call (RPC) An application-level interface used by programmers in the development of distributed programs. RPC services used RPC to support Active Directory replication traffic.

Replay attack Occurs when attackers use a protocol analyzer to capture packets as they move across the network. Once the attackers have the packets on their machine, they can extract the packets that contain, modify them, and then place them back on the network.

Repudiation This type of threat represents the risk that a legitimate transaction will be disowned by one of the participants. Repudiation is an element of the STRIDE acronym.

Revocation Invalidating a certificate before it expires.

Risk The possibility of suffering a loss, and the extent of damage that would result if the loss occurs.

Risk analysis Identifying and determining the perceived value of assets, should damage occur.

Risk management Identifying risks, analyzing the risks, and creating a plan to manage them.

Risk management plan A plan for identifying and prioritizing assets, justifying security costs, and identifying threats.

Risk statement Identifying a threat and determining the impact should it occur.

Rivest Cipher #4 (RC4) algorithm A symmetric key algorithm designed by Ron Rivest or RSA Security. It is a pseudo-random number generator (PSAG) initialized from a secret key. A PSAG is an algorithm that, when run, generates a sequence of numbers that are independent.

Rivest, Shamir, Adleman (RSA) Asymmetric algorithm developed by Ron Rivest, Adi Shamir, and Leonard Adleman from the Massachusetts Institute of Technology in 1977. It can be used for key exchange, encryption/decryption and digital signatures. It is the most public key algorithm in use today with implementations in Secure Sockets Layer (SSL) protocol, Secure Electronic Transactions (SET) and Pretty Good Privacy (PGP) as well as other cryptographic authentication and messaging schemes.

Rogue wireless access points (WAPs) WAPs that operate without the company's authorization.

Root CA The most trusted Certification Authority (CA) in a CA hierarchy.

RSA See Rivest, Shamir, Adleman.

SAC See Special Administration Console.

SACL See System access control list.

Schema partition/naming context Contains definitions of all the objects that can be created in Active Directory and their associated attributes. This partition is replicated to all domain controllers in the entire forest.

Screened subnet A network that sits between a private (trusted) network and a public network, such as the Internet, that is not trusted. It is also known as a demilitarized zone (DMZ) network.

Secedit.exe A command-line utility that performs the same functions as the Security Configuration and Analysis snap-in. It differs in that it can be called from a batch file or script and enables you to apply specific security configurations in a template.

Secure Hash Algorithm-1 Algorithm used to provide data integrity when using Authentication Header and Encapsulating Security Protocol. It is required when a company must adhere to Federal Information Processing Standards (FIPS) regulations.

Secure Sockets Layer (SSL) A protocol developed by Netscape that encrypts communications over the Internet, protects against modification of packets, and ensures the information is sent to the intended server. Used frequently by e-commerce sites to protect consumer credit card information.

Security awareness program Includes communicating management guidelines regarding the protection of company assets to employees and guidelines; ongoing security awareness training; making sure employees understand the reasoning behind security controls; and training employees to recognize when intrusions occur, how to report them and what actions to take to reduce damage.

Security boundary Define the area for which an administrator's security authority does not cross.

Security Configuration and Analysis (SCA) snap-in A tool that can be used to configure security settings on a local computer by using security templates. It also provides the ability to analyze the current security configuration of the computer and compare it against settings contained in a security template.

Security descriptor Contains information such as the object's owner, a discretionary access control list (DACL), and a system access control list (SACL).

Security identifier (SID) An alphanumeric structure that is issued when the object is created and is used to uniquely identify a user, group, or computer.

Security levels Settings in a Software Restriction Policy that decides whether all software may run or none may do so. These settings are referred to as Unrestricted and Disallowed, respectively.

Security patch A fix that has been released by Microsoft to address a security-related vulnerability in a specific product. Also known as a security update.

Security policy A high-level plan of how management expects security to be practiced within the company. It defines what actions are deemed acceptable by employees, how security will be implemented and followed, and the consequences for not complying.

Security policy boundary Defines areas where a security policy can be implemented and enforced.

Security principals Users and groups included in discretionary access control lists (DACLs) and system access control lists (SACLs).

Security procedures Written documents that provide step-by-step instructions on how the security policy is implemented.

Security reference monitor (SRM) Operating system component responsible for creating and attaching security descriptors to objects. Checks user token SIDs against SIDs in DACL to determine level of authorization.

Security template A collection of security configuration settings that are stored as a text file using the *.inf* extension.

Security template snap-in A tool that can be used both to create new security templates as well as modify existing templates. Primarily it provides a single location where you can manage all existing security attributes.

Segmenting The process of dividing a network into separate physical or logical parts using devices, such as firewalls, proxy servers, and/or routers.

Selective authentication The ability to limit authentication across a trust.

Serial Port Console Redirection (SPCR) table Read by EMS during the installation process. Provides information on how the firmware and the service processor use ports specified for out-of-band management.

Server Side Includes (SSI) Extension used to centrally manage updates to multiple Web pages. It is used in situations where the same content appears on multiple Web pages throughout a Web site.

Service pack An update or fix that recognizes issues and makes them available to customers. These issues are discovered by customers or by an internal testing group at Microsoft and address areas such as overall system reliability, compatibility issues with applications, security and/or setup issues.

Service processors Provide a way to manage a computer using out-of band connections without use of the operating system. They typically come as part of a PCI card or integrated into the computer's system board.

Service Set Identifier (SSID) The name used to identify a wireless network.

Service ticket (TGS) A ticket issued by the Ticket Granting Service. The client presents the ticket to the requested network service to provide the user's identity to the service and the service's identity to the user.

Shadow Copies of Shared Folders A previous version of the file or folder at a specific point in time. Shadow Copies of Shared Folders is a new feature in Windows Server 2003.

Share permissions Set of permissions that restricts access to shared folders, and files and folders within that folder, on a network. Cannot be applied to individual files.

Shared key authentication Provides authentication through the use of a shared secret.

Shared passphrase Password or phrase that is known to two parties. Must be distributed via secure channels.

Shortcut trust A type of trust that can be implemented to reduce the length of the trust path and improve authentication performance between domains.

SID See Security identifier.

SID filtering The process of not allowing SIDs to be used outside of the forest.

Simple Mail Transfer Protocol (SMTP) A protocol used to send e-mail between two servers.

Simple Mail Transfer Protocol (SMTP) service Uses SMTP to provide mail delivery services. It can be used to provide e-mail services on Web servers for Web applications.

Single loss expectancy (SLE) The amount of money lost should a risk occur one time.

Single sign-on (SSO) Allows network users to access all authorized network resources, on the basis of a single authentication credential.

Sites Used by Active Directory to determine which IP subnets are considered to have good connection rates. It assumes that IP subnets within a site are well connected and that bandwidth is freely available.

Slave DNS Server A DNS server that receives its zone information from another DNS server.

Smart card enrollment station Advanced version of the Web Enrollment Support pages. It enables a security principal to act as an enrollment agent on behalf of another user.

SMS See Systems Management Server.

SMTP See Simple Mail Transfer Protocol.

SMTP relay The process of one system's contacting a mail server to send e-mail to other systems the standard e-mail protocols.

Sniffer program A program that intercepts packets on the network and makes their contents visible.

Sniffing Listening to another person's digital or voice communications. Sometimes called eavesdropping.

Software Restriction Policies Policies that allow you to identify and specify what software is allowed to run.

Software Restriction Rules Used to determine the conditions under which an application will be allowed or not allowed to run.

Software Update Services (SUS) A free Windows Server add-on that enables small and mid-sized businesses to handle patch management for servers and clients.

Spam Unsolicited, or junk, e-mail sent to many recipients to promote a service or product, sometimes bogus.

Spammer A person or company that send unsolicited, or junk, e-mail to many recipients to promote a service or product, sometimes bogus.

Special Administration Console (SAC) Command-line console used with Emergency Management Services (EMS). It enables you to restart the computer, view and end processes, set/view IP address configurations, and generate memory dump files.

Split-brain DNS A method of separating your internal and external namespaces. It is created by deploying two DNS servers. One is exposed to the Internet; the other is protected behind a firewall and is used only for internal name resolution. Also referred to as split-horizon DNS.

Spoofing A type of threat in which the attacker impersonates another user or computer. Spoofing is an element of the STRIDE acronym.

SQL See Structured Query Language.

SQL database Microsoft's multi-user relational database used for data management and analysis.

SRM See Security reference monitor.

SSI See Server Side Includes.

SSID See Service Set Identifier.

SSL See Secure Sockets Layer.

SSO See Single sign-on.

Standalone CA Stores its information in a local database as opposed to Active Directory.

State table A table in the devices memory that maintains information on current sessions.

Stateful inspection An enhanced firewall technology that provides packet filtering and also tracks the state of each session.

STRIDE A threat model designed by Michael Howard and David Leblanc. Acronym stands for Spoofing, Tampering, Repudiation, Information disclosure, Denial of Service (Dos) attack, and Elevation of privilege.

Structured Query Language (SQL) Standard interactive programming language used for getting information from and updating a relational database.

Subauthentication A mechanism used by IIS to synchronize passwords stored in the local security accounts database or in Active Directory. Although subauthentication was enabled by default for IIS 5 and earlier, it is disabled in IIS 6.0 to address a security vulnerability that arises when the administrator of a Web site gives the anonymous user elevated privileges without providing a corresponding password.

Subordinate CA Issues certificates only to issuing CAs when a three-level hierarchy is designed. Also known as an intermediary CA.

SubWeb A part of a FrontPage Web. It resembles a subdirectory and is kept separate from the rest of the Web. SubWebs typically are implemented for areas of a Web site that do not have interrelated topics.

Supplicant A wireless client device that is attempting to authenticate with a wireless access point (WAP).

SUS See Software Update Services.

SUS hierarchy A collection of SUS servers that function in a parent-child relationship.

Symmetric key cryptography Involves the use of a common secret or private key that both security principals must use to secure their communications.

SysAdmin, Audit, Network, Security (SANS) Institute Develops, maintains, and makes available the largest collection of research documents about various aspects of information security and operates the Internet's early warning system, the Internet Storm Center. It was established in 1989 as a cooperative research and education organization.

System access control list (SACL) Comprised of one or more access control entries (ACEs), enables administrators to log attempts to access the object.

Systems Management Server (SMS) Includes wizards for packaging and deploying security updates and software installations. SMS is used for large organizations that need greater platform support and more control over their security updates than SUS can provide.

SYSVOL A shared directory that stores the server copy of the domain's public files that must be shared for common access and replication throughout the domain. It contains information such as user/computer logon scripts and Group Policy information.

Tampering A type of threat in which a user maliciously modifies data. Tampering is an element of the STRIDE acronym.

Tape libraries A device that contains multiple tape drives that can have many tape slots. Uses a robot that automatically swaps tapes as they fill.

Tape vaulting The process of transferring backup media by courier.

Telnet Enables a remote user to log on to the computer and use the command line to run console programs.

Terminal concentrators Provides a single networked interface that enables you to view data on multiple servers that use serial ports for their out-of-band communication.

Terminal emulator A terminal emulator is basically a window that emulates a particular type of terminal to interact with EMS.

Terminal Server A computer running Terminal Services that provides a way to distribute Windows-based programs with a network server.

Terminal Services Can be used as a remote administration tool.

TGS Ticket Granting Service.

TGT Ticket Granting Ticket.

Threat A danger or vulnerability to an asset.

Threat model A model used to identifying potential threats to assets.

Ticket cache An area of memory protected by the Local Security Authority (LSA). This area of memory is never paged to disk. All tickets and keys stored here are destroyed when the user logs off.

Ticket Granting Service (TGS) Issues tickets for a desired service, which are in turn given to users for access to the service. The service usually runs on the same computer as the Key Distribution Center (KDC).

Ticket Granting Ticket (TGT) A ticket that enables a Kerberos client to obtain additional tickets without applying for them from the Key Distribution Center (KDC).

Transitive trust A trust that extends between multiple domains.

Triple DES (3DES) Developed by IBM, 3DES was invented to improve security over DES by applying DES encryption three times. It uses a 192-bit key as input and breaks it down into three 64-bit keys

Trojan horse A program with code that appears harmless but is malicious. Unlike viruses, Trojan horses do not replicate themselves. For them to spread, you must invite them onto your computer—e.g., open an e-mail attachment or download an unfamiliar.

Truck vaulting The process of transferring backup media by courier.

Trust model Represents the number of trusts within and between domains and forests.

Trust path The path an authentication attempt takes between parent-child domain relationships.

Trust relationship Allows a user in one forest/domain to gain access to resources in another forest/domain.

Two-factor authentication A form of multifactor authentication in which two factors are used to authenticate a user. The options include something the user is, something the user knows, and something the user has.

Two-way initiated connection This occurs when either router can perform the role of a calling or answering router.

USAPA See USA Patriot Act.

Uniform resource locator (URL) Address of a site on the Internet or a file on a Web server.

Uniting and Strengthening America by Providing Appropriate Tools Required to Intercept and Obstruct Terrorism Act of 2001, U.S.A. PATRIOT Act (USAPA) Legislation established to address terrorism acts after September 11, 2001. Enables government agencies to monitor oral, wire, and electronic communications.

Universal Naming Convention (UNC) authentication A mechanism that can be used when users need to be authenticated while accessing a Web site or virtual directory whose content is stored in a remote share. This is accomplished by using a preconfigured account, specified by the administrator, which has permissions to the remote resource. Also known as passthrough authentication.

Universally unique identifier (UUID) A distinct number assigned to a Remote Procedure Call (RPC) service upon startup. When the RPC service obtains a port number, it registers it with the UUID in the computer's Registry.

UUID See Universally unique identifier.

Validity period The start and end of time period in which a certificate is intended to be used.

Virtual directory Directory that is not located in your home directory but appears to users as though it were.

Virtual private network (VPN) Networks that enable you to use the Internet or other public carriers as a transit for private network traffic, usually in encrypted form.

Virus A small program written to alter the way a computer operates, without the permission or knowledge of the user. It executes and replicates itself by copying itself to an executable file.

Vision statement Provides insight as to what a company wants to accomplish over a period of time.

Voluntary tunnel This type of tunnel is created when a VPN client initiates a connection to a VPN server. It is considered voluntary because the client must initiate the actual connection.

VPN See Virtual private network.

VPN accelerator card Cards that offload encryption operations from the computer's processor to a dedicated one on the card itself.

WAP See Wireless Access Point.

War driving The process of using Global Positioning Satellite (GPS) receivers to map areas of a city that are using access points and identifies which ones are secured.

Web Enrollment Support pages Web pages used to enroll and renew certificates.

WEP See Wired Equivalent Privacy.

Whoami Utility that enables you to view the contents of an access token.

Wi-Fi Alliance A non-profit international organization formed in 1999 to certify interoperability of wireless LAN products based on IEEE 802.11 standards.

WiFi Protected Access (WPA) An interim version of 802.11i that was widely implemented in operating systems and devices in 2003 by the Wi-Fi Alliance who could not wait for 802.11i to be ratified.

Windows authentication When selected as the method of authentication, the RRAS server uses either its local security accounts database or a domain account database.

Windows Installer package A file that containing all of the information required to install or uninstall a program. It is used by Windows Installer, a component of the Windows operating system.

Windows Logo Program A Microsoft program that ensures the applications that receive the "Designed for Windows" logo have passed Windows compatibility testing.

Windows Media Player Software that enables you to play and organize digital media files on the computer and the Internet.

Windows Server 2003 forest functional level A Windows Server 2003 functional level that requires all domain controllers to run the Window Server 2003 operating system.

Windows Update A consumer Web site, run by Microsoft, that provides critical updates, security fixes, and software downloads.

Windows Zero Configuration service (WZCSVC) Available in Windows XP; used to dynamically select a wireless network to which to attempt connection. The wireless network adapter and its Network Driver Interface Specification (NDIS) driver must support this service for it to function.

Wired Equivalent Privacy (WEP) A security protocol for wireless LANs defined in the original IEEE 802.11 standards.

Wireless access filter A filter list on a wireless access point that is used to control access based on the media access control list.

Wireless access point (WAP) A device that connects wireless clients together. Typically used to connect wireless clients to a wired network.

Wireless local area network (WLAN) Functions by sending radio signals that are broadcast over the airwaves using certain radio frequency (RF) ranges (2.4 GHz - 5.875 GHz, depending upon the wireless standard implemented). Signals pass through not only walls inside the corporate office building, but also an exterior wall into an adjacent parking lot or street. They also can pass through floors of multi-story buildings. A WLAN offers mobility, convenience, and greater flexibility in contrast to wired LANs. However, they raise additional security concerns that network administrators must address.

World Wide Web Publishing service Must be running to provide Web connectivity and administration through the IIS Manager.

Worm A program that replicates itself from computer to computer without the use of a host file. This differs from viruses, which require the spreading of a host file to replicate.

WPA See WiFi Protected Access.

WZCSVC See Windows Zero Configuration service.

X.509 standard The most widely used standard for defining the contents of digital certificates.

Zone transfers Used to update zone records on secondary DNS servers.

Exam 70-298 Objectives

Creating the Conceptual Design for Network Infrastructure Security by Gathering and Analyzing Business and Technical Requirements

1.01 Analyze business requirements for designing security. Considerations include existing policies and procedures, sensitivity of data, cost, legal requirements, end-user impact, interoperability, maintainability, scalability, and risk.

- 1.01 (a) Analyze existing security policies and procedures.
- 1.01 (b) Analyze the organizational requirements for securing data.
- 1.01 (c) Analyze the security requirements of different types of data.
- 1.01 (d) Analyze risks to security within the current IT administration structure and security practices.

1.02 Design a framework for designing and implementing security. The framework should include prevention, detection, isolation, and recovery.

- 1.02 (a) Predict threats to your network from internal and external sources.
- 1.02 (b) Design a process for responding to incidents.
- 1.02 (c) Design segmented networks.
- 1.02 (d) Design a process for recovering services.

1.03 Analyze technical constraints when designing security.

- 1.03 (a) Identify capabilities of the existing infrastructure.
- 1.03 (b) Identify technology limitations.
- 1.03 (c) Analyze interoperability constraints.

Creating the Logical Design for Network Infrastructure Security

2.01 Design a public key infrastructure (PKI) that uses Certificate Services.

- 2.01 (a) Design a certification authority (CA) hierarchy implementation. Types include geographical, organizational, and trusted.
- 2.01 (b) Design enrollment and distribution processes.
- 2.01 (c) Establish renewal, revocation and auditing processes.
- 2.01 (d) Design security for CA servers.

2.02 Design a logical authentication strategy.

- 2.02 (a) Design certificate distribution.
- 2.02 (b) Design forest and domain trust models.
- 2.02 (c) Design security that meets interoperability requirements.
- 2.02 (d) Establish account and password requirements for security.

2.03 Design security for network management.

- 2.03 (a) Manage the risk of managing networks.
- 2.03 (b) Design the administration of servers by using common administration tools. Tools include Microsoft Management Console (MMC), Terminal Server, Remote Desktop for Administration, Remote Assistance, and Telnet.
- 2.03 (c) Design security for Emergency Management Services.

2.04 Design a security update infrastructure.

- 2.04 (a) Design a Software Update Services (SUS) infrastructure.
- 2.04 (b) Design Group Policy to deploy software updates.
- 2.04 (c) Design a strategy for identifying computers that are not at the current patch level.

Creating the Physical Design for Network Infrastructure Security

3.01 Design network infrastructure security.

- 3.01 (a) Specify the required protocols for a firewall configuration.
- 3.01 (b) Design IP filtering.
- 3.01 (c) Design an IPSec policy.
- 3.01 (d) Secure a DNS implementation.
- 3.01 (e) Design security for data transmission.

3.02 Design security for wireless networks.

- 3.02 (a) Design public and private wireless LANs.
- 3.02 (b) Design 802.1x authentication for wireless networks.

Exam 70-298 Objectives (cont'd)

3.03 Design user authentication for Internet Information Services (IIS).
- 3.03 (a) Design user authentication for a Web site by using certificates.
- 3.03 (b) Design user authentication for a Web site by using IIS authentication.
- 3.03 (c) Design user authentication for a Web site by using RADIUS for IIS authentication.

3.04 Design security for Internet Information Services (IIS).
- 3.04 (a) Design security for Web sites that have different technical requirements by enabling only the minimum required services.
- 3.04 (b) Design a monitoring strategy for IIS.
- 3.04 (c) Design an IIS baseline that is based on business requirements.
- 3.04 (d) Design a content management strategy for updating an IIS server.

3.05 Design security for communication between networks.
- 3.05 (a) Select protocols for VPN access.
- 3.05 (b) Design VPN connectivity.
- 3.05 (c) Design demand-dial routing between internal networks.

3.06 Design security for communication with external organizations.
- 3.06 (a) Design an extranet infrastructure.
- 3.06 (b) Design a strategy for cross-certification of Certificate Services.

3.07 Design security for servers that have specific roles. Roles include domain controller, network infrastructure server, file server, IIS server, terminal server, and POP3 mail server.
- 3.07 (a) Define a baseline security template for all systems.
- 3.07 (b) Create a plan to modify baseline security templates according to role.

Designing an Access Control Strategy for Data

4.01 Design an access control strategy for directory services.
- 4.01 (a) Create a delegation strategy.
- 4.01 (b) Analyze auditing requirements.
- 4.01 (c) Design the appropriate group strategy for accessing resources.
- 4.01 (d) Design a permission structure for directory service objects.

4.02 Design an access control strategy for files and folders.
- 4.02 (a) Design a strategy for the encryption and decryption of files and folders.
- 4.02 (b) Design a permission structure for files and folders.
- 4.02 (c) Design security for a backup and recovery strategy.
- 4.02 (d) Analyze auditing requirements.

4.03 Design an access control strategy for the registry.
- 4.03 (a) Design a permission structure for registry objects.
- 4.03 (b) Analyze auditing requirements.

Creating the Physical Design for Client Infrastructure Security

5.01 Design a client authentication strategy.
- 5.01 (a) Analyze authentication requirements.
- 5.01 (b) Establish account and password security requirements.

5.02 Design a security strategy for client remote access.
- 5.02 (a) Design remote access policies.
- 5.02 (b) Design access to internal resources.
- 5.02 (c) Design an authentication provider and accounting strategy for remote network access by using Internet Authentication Service (IAS).

5.03 Design a strategy for securing client computers. Considerations include desktop and portable computers.
- 5.03 (a) Design a strategy for hardening client operating systems.
- 5.03 (b) Design a strategy for restricting user access to operating system features.